For Margaret —

6 —
Scan

D0395908

From There To Here

Stories of Adjustment to Spinal Cord Injury

Edited by Gary Karp and Stanley D. Klein, Ph.D.

No Limits Communications, Inc.

Publication of this book made possible by a grant from
Independence Technology, a Johnson & Johnson company

Published by
No Limits Communications
P.O. Box 220
Horsham, PA 19044
888-850-0344
www.newmobility.com

Library of Congress Control Number: 2003116411

ISBN 0-9712842-2-9

Printed in the United States of America

From There To Here

Stories of Adjustment to Spinal Cord Injury

Edited by Gary Karp and Stanley D. Klein, Ph.D.

No Limits Communications, Inc.

Publication of this book made possible by a grant from
Independence Technology, a Johnson & Johnson company

Contents

Contents

Contents

Acknowledgements

———⦻———

We sincerely thank our publisher, Jeff Leonard, for his immediate enthusiasm for this book from the moment we proposed it, to Jean Dobbs for her guidance and professionalism as managing editor, and to Patti Fitzpatrick for her graphics skills in creating this excellent layout. Much appreciation also to essay author, Ginger Lane for the cover photos.

We deeply appreciate the support of Independence Technology, a Johnson & Johnson company, whose underwriting of this book will help it to reach so many more people who will benefit from its insights.

Gary would like to express his appreciation to his wife, Paula Siegel, for her absolute support and love, his writers' group, Mark Johnson and Peter Winchell, his family, and Oscar Ichazo. Stan thanks Meredith Ellis for her continuing support and Sarah Klein for her typing skills.

A Word From Our Sponsor

———— ∞∞∞ ————

Independence Technology, L.L.C. is proud to be a partner in the publication of *From There to Here: Stories of Adjustment to Spinal Cord Injury*. We believe our support of this book reflects our vision as a partner and advocate of people with disabilities and our mission to provide products and services that increase their independence. We are part of the Johnson & Johnson family of companies and share a longstanding belief that our first responsibility is to be of service to health care professionals, nurses, consumers, mothers, fathers, and all others who use our products.

Whether you are an individual who has recently become disabled, the friend or family member of such an individual, or perhaps someone who simply needs a little encouragement, we believe that you will find the stories contained in this book insightful, informative, inspiring, and comforting. These are our sole objectives in sponsoring this important resource; Independence Technology, L.L.C. is not responsible for the content, nor are we sharing in the proceeds from the sales of this book.

You will discover through these personal essays that regardless of your current circumstances and how uncertain the future may seem, you are not alone. Because these are the autobiographies of individuals whose lives were suddenly changed as a result of a spinal cord injury, we realize that there may be language or subject matter content that some readers consider disturbing or inappropriate. However, these stories were written to express the denial, anger, depression, and fear — or whatever feelings we may experience — when our lifestyles are suddenly interrupted by a life-changing event. Such language is the natural expression of some of the voices speaking so honestly and openly in these pages with the generous intention of helping others.

What we find most inspirational about these stories — by people of all ages and all walks of life — are their varied journeys back to active and meaningful living following their injuries. They are not simply survivors. And though their lifestyles and careers may have changed, what matters — and what we celebrate — is the richness of the lives they live today.

Foreword

————⦵⦵⦵————

By Marcie Roth,
Executive Director, National Spinal Cord Injury Association

Y ou — or someone you care about — is "There." They are dealing with the initial onslaught of a spinal cord trauma. You're probably wondering how in the world anyone gets to "Here."

"There" begins in an emergency room or hospital bed when a person learns that she/he has a spinal cord injury (SCI) or disease. It's a time that evokes a massive reconsideration of one's life and future — perhaps one's very identity. It is an experience of great change, often of confusion and pain — physical, emotional, and spiritual.

"Here" is where people lead a successful, fulfilling life with the effects of their SCI. "Here" is a place they could not have imagined from "There." It is a place of active living, in which their SCI is integrated into how they move through their lives, with a clear sense of who they are — with, and entirely apart from, their disability.

As Executive Director of the National Spinal Cord Injury Association (NSCIA), and as an active member of the disability community for more than thirty years, I have come to know many people who have traveled from "There" to "Here." Gary Karp is one of them.

When I first met Gary in 1998, he was about to publish his important book, *Life On Wheels: For The Active Wheelchair User* (O'Reilly & Associates, 1999), a vehicle for him to share insights from his own disability experience with other wheelchair users, their family members and friends, and the professionals who serve them. With this new book, Gary and his co-editor, Stanley D. Klein, have added another valuable resource to the set of tools available to help people make the best possible transition from "There" to "Here."

At NSCIA, our mission is to educate and empower survivors of spinal cord injury and disease to achieve and maintain the highest levels of independence, health, and personal fulfillment. We have seen the power of quality information towards these ends. We have also seen how experienced people with SCI, like the writers in this book, are effective models of the potential to move through and transcend the impacts of sudden trauma.

Hope for a rich, full life is a motivator. But hope based only on desire risks unrealistic expectations. Hope based on real examples translates into real goals. There is assurance in seeing that people just like you have done what feels impossible — "If they did it, why can't I?" Such is the source of the empowerment offered by this book.

The stories you are about to read demonstrate the many different ways in which people adapt to — and make peace with — the realities of life with a disability. The essay authors have courageously shared intimate details about their struggles and their joys, their problems and methods, as they learned how to respond to environmental as well as attitudinal barriers while continuing to grow in their personal, professional, and spiritual lives.

Such is the power of peer support, the core stuff of what we do at NSCIA. Many staff members at our Resource Center (800-962-9629; www.spinalcord.org) have personal experience with SCI, and we work hard to connect individuals with one another via our extensive Chapter and Support Group Network.

These essay authors are not superstars or martyrs. They are real women and men who live real lives in communities throughout the United States and Canada. They work, travel, have fun, have friends, and are sexual. At NSCIA we have seen beyond a doubt that this is far more the rule than the exception for people with spinal cord injury and disease. We are very pleased to see that the community of people with SCI have access to this very valuable and intimate new look into the journeys of people who have made the trip from There to Here.

Marcie Roth
Washington, D.C.

Introduction

———— ∞∞∞∞ ————

A Montana lineman, a Native American woman, a wounded Vietnam veteran, a skinny dipper, an auto mechanic, a teenager working a summer job on a farm, a Japanese student, an Explorer Scout learning about law enforcement, and an elementary school music teacher. These are just some of the diverse people who share their experiences in this book. In their own way, each one faced the process of adjusting to a spinal cord injury (SCI) and its many implications in their lives.

In their essays, they share their pride at having found their own way through the initial trauma, their struggle with sudden and substantial life changes, and their arrival at something they consider "adjustment." All agree that the process is lifelong and that their SCI experience has been a rich source of discovery about themselves.

The period immediately following a spinal cord injury is overwhelming — for the person with paralysis as well as for family and friends. It is a time of powerful emotions in which the routine of daily life has been thrown off track, and one faces a new and unfamiliar array of tasks and decisions. Most confounding, the future is a mystery. What will life be like for everyone involved? What are the options for the person using wheels instead of legs for mobility? What dreams and plans have to be surrendered? Can new dreams replace them? These are intimidating questions. Anyone would feel hard-pressed to imagine how to deal with them — much less thrive and live happily with paralysis.

The essay authors are ordinary ("normal"), everyday women and men who, on the mysterious journey of spinal cord injury, chose life over surrender. Contrary to media stereotypes that only superhuman, heroic people succeed in the context of disability, these very real people have used their resources and talents as best they can, and have moved on to reclaim their lives — and more.

They tell it like it is — without sugarcoating. They show us the fears, doubts, and obstacles on their journeys — and they celebrate their satisfactions and surprising breakthroughs.

How It All Began

This book was conceived in a restaurant near Harvard Square in Cambridge, Massachusetts. Gary was in town on a speaking date, and the Boston area is Stan's home turf.

Stan had a recent success with a book of essays called *You Will Dream New Dreams: Inspiring Personal Stories by Parents of Children with Disabilities* (Kensington Books, 2001). Aware of the success of Gary's book, *Life On Wheels: For the Active Wheelchair User* (O'Reilly & Associates, 1999), and his nearly thirty years of personal experience with SCI, Stan asked whether a similar book of essays could be useful for people with SCI and their loved ones.

Gary described how most people with a recent SCI that he meets want to know two things. "They ask me how I got from 'there' (recently injured) to 'here' (fulfilling life), and how long it took. We can ask people to focus on their own process of adjustment rather than merely giving advice. Then, readers will pick up on the parts of the stories that are relevant to their own lives."

After a conversation with Jeff Leonard — publisher of *New Mobility* magazine — and a draft essay by Gary, *From There To Here* was under way. Full-page ads inviting people to submit an essay appeared in *New Mobility*, and the guidelines were spread via the Internet. After sorting through many thoughtful and moving essays, Gary and Stan selected forty-four and went to work with the authors.

We encouraged the authors to reach deeply into their inner thoughts and feelings and to lay out the darkness, so as to emphasize the light they ultimately reached. We did this because we believe it is important to share emotions, sorrows, and joys with loved ones, friends, and/or trusted professionals — and to enable readers to feel a personal connection with the authors.

The questions addressed in these essays loom largest in the first stages of the SCI experience, yet we believe that there is much to discover here for anyone at any point along the path of life with a spinal cord injury, even those who are well past the initial trauma of SCI.

A Brief Spinal Cord Primer

For readers not yet familiar with the levels of spinal cord injury and their implications, here is a brief primer.

The higher the location of a trauma to the spinal cord, the more of the body is disconnected from communication with the brain. "Messages" that originate in the brain travel down the spinal cord, and then branch off from the cord to the peripheral nerves to stimulate the muscles to move. Sensory "messages" travel up to the brain via the cord. The spinal cord and the brain are referred to as the central nervous system.

The spinal cord, which is like a cable made up of many wires, is surrounded by a column of bones called vertebrae, which make up the spine. The top section of the column, consisting of seven vertebrae in the neck, is called the cervical (abbreviated as C) section. The second section of the column, consisting of twelve vertebrae corresponding to the rib cage, is called the thoracic (T) section. The third section, consisting of five vertebrae in the lower back, is called the lumbar (L) section. Each vertebra within each of the three sections is numbered. Accordingly, the shorthand for an injury to the third vertebra in the cervical section is C3. When two numbers are used (e.g., C3-4), two vertebrae were impacted. Throughout this book — and the everyday language of rehabilitation — injury levels are described in these terms.

When an injury is high up in the neck, most of the body is disconnected from conscious control. People with cervical injuries are considered "quadriplegic" or "tetraplegic," a term the medical community sometimes uses. At the highest level, a "quad" might be unable to use his hands or arms, and possibly rely on a ventilator for breathing support, unable to contract his diaphragm muscles to expand his lungs.

When an injury is below the cervical level, the person is able to use his arms and hands and is considered "paraplegic." Most people with spinal cord injuries also experience impairment of their bowel and bladder functions and loss of some sexual response.

The term "severed" is sometimes used to describe spinal cord injuries, but in fact the cord is rarely severed. The majority of SCIs are "compression" injuries, in which blood flowing to the cord is stopped for a long enough period of time to cause cell death in the "axons," which carry the messages to the nerve endings. This disconnects the flow of messages to and from that area of the body and below.

Medical texts display topographic maps of the body indicating which areas are affected at a given level of injury. In actual practice, these are often inaccurate because any two people with a given level of injury are likely to have different degrees of actual motor and sensory impairment.

Approximately half of all spinal cord injuries are considered "incomplete." This means that some muscle and/or sensory functions exist below the level of the injury. Some people with SCI are able to stand, and some can even walk. Occasionally, people make a full recovery from a spinal cord trauma. Over time, everyone finds out for themselves what their injury means to their own body — and in their lives.

Categorizing people by their level is dangerous because people may believe that their level of injury defines specific expectations for their degree of ability and function. A paraplegic doesn't necessarily have a better life or more abilities than a quadriplegic. This book illustrates that level does not — on its own — predict quality of a life lived with SCI. To emphasize that level does not indicate quality of life, we have not organized the essays by level of injury.

Although each essay opens with some "demographics" — level of injury, date of injury, age at injury, and hometown — we urge readers to take the level with a grain of salt — and read on. Any essay author, regardless of level of injury, may provide that particular spark of understanding that can make a difference for someone who is trying to find his way. Readers should feel free to read the essays in any order.

The question of recovery looms large in the minds of anyone with a recent SCI, as well as family and friends. People do not generally make a full recovery from a spinal cord injury because the cells in the central nervous system cannot regenerate in response to trauma (in contrast to nerves outside of the central nervous system that can). Partial recovery is, however, quite common. Some initial impairment can be associated with shock to the cord, rather than actual structural damage. Some people make surprising recoveries that could not have been predicted.

While our essay writers would rather not have these particular stories to tell, they are not waiting around for a cure. They are interested in and generally support the research — one is himself a researcher — and will welcome any discoveries that would benefit them. In the meantime, they have chosen to get out and live their lives.

Our Hopes for This Book

This collection of rich, human stories can shed light on the uncharted path ahead. When the light at the end of the tunnel is not in view, it can be discouraging and frustrating as one tries to discern which way to turn. We are confident that anyone dealing with an SCI experience — both people who are recently injured as well as people who are some years "post-injury" — will find something in this collection that will resonate, connect, and provide hope that what feels impossible today may not necessarily be so tomorrow.

Individuals with spinal cord injuries have a great deal in common and are a unique group of human beings, yet their needs and desires are the same as those without SCI. By telling their own stories and listening to the stories of others, they can be both teachers and learners. They teach from the their unique awareness of how adaptable we humans are, and they learn because they know the value of confronting change and being open to its lessons.

Certain themes arise throughout the essays:

• A spinal cord injury doesn't just happen to an individual — it happens to family, friends, and community. The love and support of family, friends, and community can make a meaningful difference in how the journey of SCI is experienced.

• People with SCI find out that people will stick around even when you are depressed, angry, and/or rude. They also find out who their friends are — the true ones stick around when the going gets tough. Sadly, some don't.

• The wide range of difficult and painful emotions people experience is a normal part of the SCI experience. The feelings do not last forever. There is sadness; some dreams are lost, new dreams are created. People need to mourn their losses, as these stories of healing demonstrate. By honestly expressing our emotions with loved ones, we can comfort and gain strength from one another. While there are no easy answers, people find ways to cope and discover inner resources they did not imagine existed.

• Peer counseling programs and self-help groups are a very helpful part of the rehabilitation process. Healing takes place far beyond the physical plane, encompassing the emotional and spiritual. In such groups, people discover they are not alone in their emotions and fears. They share practical wisdom, and can challenge denial. While *From There To Here* is like a peer support group in a book, it is no substitute for real, personal interaction.

• Unfortunately, emotional and spiritual needs are sometimes not given high priority by health professionals or insurance providers. Yet, when these needs are neglected, the healing process becomes far more expensive in both human and financial terms. For example, when an individual loses the ability to walk, she feels sad. Feeling sad is different from feeling depressed because when that same individual is depressed, she feels that since she is unable to walk, she is worthless. Feeling worthless, she is less likely to be motivated to participate actively in her own rehabilitation, requiring longer support services, and risking expensive secondary health problems. Individuals who are depressed can benefit from clinical treatment.

• In the "outside" world, both environmental and attitudinal barriers can restrict people with disabilities. When people with disabilities believe societal prejudices about people with disabilities, they may lower their own expectations and misperceive themselves. The language widely used to describe disability aggravates the problem. People who think of themselves as "confined" to a wheelchair are more likely to buy into a negative self-image. At the other extreme, believing that one needs to "overcome" disability raises the bar to a heroic level, when, in fact, people who get the services and support they need typically succeed with SCI. They "adapt" to their disability.

• The journey never ends. Today's "Here" becomes tomorrow's "There."

With deep regrets we note that Vickie Baker, one of our authors, died of natural causes in October 2003. We struggled with the question of how to note Vickie's loss because we were concerned that it might suggest that spinal cord injury shortens one's life span. There is no statistical basis for such an assertion — quite the contrary. People with spinal cord injuries who maintain their health can look forward to living a normal life span. We honor Vickie's memory with the treasured contribution she made to these pages.

We have been honored and deeply moved by the willingness of the essay writers to share their very personal reflections. We have been energized by the courage and wisdom they offer out of a desire for their life experiences to offer meaning and insight to others. We appreciate their wonderful efforts.

Gary Karp & Stanley D. Klein

Falling Into Grace

Elizabeth Fetter Eastman
T4-5
Age at SCI: 17
Date of SCI: August 22, 1965
St. Paul, Minnesota

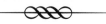

*F*ifteen or so years ago I stopped using the word "accident" to describe that defining moment in 1965 when I became paraplegic. These days, I say, "I injured myself." I was a participant in the choices that led to my climbing a sixty-foot Douglas Fir. I chose to ignore my gut telling me, "This is dangerous," as I pawed through the thick, dead, lower branches to find the trunk. And I chose to stay there as it got dark. Then, climbing down, I stepped on a dead branch, and fell forty feet.

I was an athletic seventeen-year-old, but insecure and wanting to fit in, even though I was captain of the high school tennis team. As a counselor in training at a tennis camp situated at the foot of the White Mountains in New Hampshire, I had caved in to peer pressure and climbed an unsafe tree while playing a game of "counselor hunt." Now, when people ask how I came to be using this wheelchair, my answering with a passive word like "accident" feels like a small but meaningful erosion of my soul.

When I landed from my fall, I was still conscious, but in shock. I was taken to Dartmouth's Mary Hitchcock Hospital for surgery to relieve the pressure on my spine. I had not been in a hospital since I was born.

When our retired family minister came to visit me, I knew this was serious. In my childhood he was the very icon of authority, standing high above us in the ornately carved pulpit. Now antiseptic white walls surrounded us and my hospital bed took up seventy-five percent of the room. As he leaned against my bedrail, he greeted me in his deep, authoritative voice.

"Hello, Dr. Van Dyke," I replied softly. Every word was an effort, yet even the unnamable feelings clambering up inside me like unruly toddlers could not override my well-learned manners. We visited briefly and then he held out his strong, veined hands, and asked if we could pray. As he prayed, I could feel the hotness of tears around my eyes. After he left, I cried softly. I was alone, hiding my face under the rough, starched sheets, quietly repeating the word, "Never" to myself as I pondered the forever nature of the word. Never. Walk.

That was the sum total of my grieving. True to my pattern of discounting what I intuitively knew, I didn't discuss my feelings or ask what was wrong with me, but indulged in lighthearted repartee with my white-aproned, student nurses as we read the many cards people sent me.

My mother was a large woman, often in a take-charge mode. But on these occasions, she would often come into the hospital room, look at me, and leave in tears. So I chose to be "strong for my mother," with no consciousness that my "strength" was built on a quicksand of unresolved emotions. At times I was aware of my building resentment, saying to myself, "I'm the one who is injured, and she's the one who is crying!"

After two weeks, I was flown to the Hospital of the University of Pennsylvania, near our home in suburban Philadelphia. A smiling, pear-shaped doctor spoke about my impending transfer to the rehabilitation center.

"What is a rehabilitation center?" I asked.

"A rehab center is where we will teach you to walk with braces and crutches," he said, pulling up a chair next to my bed.

"Why would I want to learn to walk with braces and crutches?"

"Well, we would hope you could walk again, but we are going to teach you to walk with braces on the assumption that you are not going to be able to walk anymore."

"Oh," I said, as I looked away from his face, and grabbed the trapeze above me to reposition myself. He put his hand over mine with a reassuring squeeze, and then left. Alone, I stared at the high pastel blue ceilings with the pipes running beneath the plaster. This time I didn't cry.

The rigorous rehabilitation program included an attempt at psychological support. I instinctively disliked the psychiatrist. I never confronted him, but I sometimes defended other patients from his verbal sparring and glared at him when he made light of emotionally difficult situations. His intellectual indictment of me included a diagnosis that I was not going through the textbook stages of grief, and he predicted that I would fall apart someday after an incident such as hitting a dog with my car.

In rehab, I learned to drive with hand controls. Not long after the psychiatrist's prediction, I was driving home from the rehab center on a weekend pass when I actually did hit and kill a dog. I was sad, but this did not trigger my unresolved pain. I was almost gleeful, thinking to myself, "See? Your prediction didn't come true."

After nine months of charming the physicians and nurses, I "graduated" from rehab. I had spent my entire senior year living at the hospital, but still graduated with my class thanks to tutors who came to visit me. The next fall I went on to a local college. At no point did I take time to emotionally adjust to my new life using a wheelchair. I got involved in wheelchair athletics, learning javelin, shot put, and discus — not out of real interest in these sports, but because they were the only athletic choices at the time. I traveled around the world to places like Germany, England, Jamaica, and Brazil, and set a record for discus.

After graduating with a B.A. in English education, I was told plainly that a person using a wheelchair would have difficulty teaching (how could one discipline a whole class?). Swayed by this advice, I chose to go to graduate school and major in counseling psychology, a field where the ratio of professional to student/client was smaller. This was the '70s, when the women's movement pooh-poohed the wife and motherhood track, urging women to pursue careers. I embraced this image, pressing forward as a single professional.

My career led me to Illinois, California, Texas, Washington, D.C., and then Minnesota. I was climbing the ladder to success. Outside, I was calm and confident. Inside, I knew I was beginning to disintegrate. I was chosen for a year in the White House Fellows program, where I was a Special Assistant to the Secretary of Transportation, Neil Goldschmidt. I stayed on working at the White House, and then was selected to be the Deputy Director for the U.N. International Year of Disabled Persons. I experienced the pleasure of saunas in Finland and coffee houses in Paris, but the undercurrent of emotional anguish still flowed beneath my cosmopolitan façade.

I was also still pushing the envelope in adventure sports. On a canoe trip with an organization that takes people of all ability levels into the wilderness, the man I was canoeing with (an epileptic) had a seizure. He fell out of our canoe, not wearing his life jacket. I slid into the water to try to save him, but he never came up. I was devastated. *This* was the "run over the dog" incident the psychiatrist had predicted, and it triggered my internal implosion. Fifteen years after my physical rehabilitation, my emotional rehabilitation had begun. At last I was going through the long-delayed stages of grief, and entered a period of depression that ebbed and flowed over the next five years.

I didn't want to stay in D.C., so I accepted a job offer from General Mills in Minneapolis. My old pattern of busy-ness was not working to keep my inner pain at bay, so — finally! — I started looking for answers in places other than my work or by moving to yet another city.

At a lecture by a woman named Anne Wilson Schaef, I heard about patterns of "addictive" living that hit so close to home that I felt she must have been a mouse in my home, observing me day and night. I was stunned to learn that all this striving — for which I had been so well rewarded — was blocking me from my neglected inner life.

To grieve the losses associated with my disability, I had to learn a whole new way of being in the world. My overanalyzing, controlling, driven self was great at stacking up achievements, but got me no closer to peace of mind. I was getting support from others to process my feelings, but I also needed to address some of the chemical imbalances that go along with depression. I believed that taking anti-depressants might offer some relief and some added ability to function, but I also thought it did not offer *healing*. I eventually landed on the doorstep of an alternative medicine practitioner.

"You are my last stop before I start on anti-depressants," I said.

"Give me four months," he answered.

I continued to do my emotional work while simultaneously detoxing with his support. As he had promised, I noticed after about four months that the sun was indeed shining and there was quite a lot to be grateful for.

I resigned from General Mills and started working as a consultant. I made enough to survive financially, while still having large chunks of time to fall apart emotionally.

At every opportunity, I participated in Anne's work called "Living In Process." Here I was finding a community of support where healing, not functioning, was the top value. I was encouraged to face the dark bramble forest, not just flee. By this time, the inner pain was so intense, that this path was clearly my best option. Gradually I was unlearning the go-getting patterns that had not gotten me anywhere I wanted to be. I was also having a whole different experience of the lower part of my body. After each massage (which I was getting weekly) I would experience a surge of aliveness energy course through me. I didn't relate to phrases like "lost the use of her legs" anymore. I was feeling supported, by my legs and trunk, by the water when I floated, by the Universe in general. Grace was finding me in the nooks and crannies of my everyday life, and I was welcoming it.

Ever so slowly I began to allow myself to accept help. I have often laughed that if God wanted someone to "get it" about asking for help, I was sure given a great set of circumstances. During my thirty-eight years as a paraplegic, I've been pregnant and have had two broken legs. Both times, I had either a baby or a small child with me. You'd think I would be a black belt at asking for help by now. Two particular experiences highlight my progress towards being able to ask for and receive help. One came before my emotional resurrection, the other after.

In the early '70s, in graduate school, our teacher asked the class to sing a song and record it. There was a raised platform in the recording studio, set up with a microphone. I sat in my wheelchair on the barren studio floor, separate from my classmates. They stood on the stage and sang. I tried to swallow the waves of hurt, but I was unable to think of how to remedy the situation.

I had learned how to ask for help around absolute necessities like carrying a heavy suitcase, but in this case I couldn't say, "Hey. I want to be part of this. Could you help me up or put the mike on the floor?"

The second experience happened about five years ago, with my four-year-old son riding on my lap at a large department store. (I got married when I was 45, and had my son at 46.) As we passed the escalator he asked, "Mom, ask someone to ride it with me!"

I hesitated.

"C'mon, Mom. You ask people for help all the time."

"Okay," I agreed. "But I need to wait for just the right person."

We waited until a woman with a light step and graying hair approached us. Her face lit up when I explained my son's desire. She took his small hand and escorted him up the escalator and then down again.

"You made my day," she said as she handed my son back to me.

"And you made ours," I smiled.

I would love to get up and walk away with all the new and life-giving ways I have learned. But today, that is not an option. Who would have thought that my struggles with my limitations would have led me to a whole new outlook on life and continually guide me to new levels of spiritual freedom and contentment? Am I grateful for these lessons? Absolutely. Would I wish that someone I love dearly, like my son, would have a similar gift? Absolutely not. I want his learning to be easy. I am not in charge of my lessons, only my reactions to them. On most days, I accept them. On my better days, I embrace them.

Elizabeth (Buffy) Fetter Eastman lives in St. Paul, Minnesota, with her husband and son. She works as a part time consultant, writer and researcher. She is active in parent activities in her son's Waldorf School. She likes exploring ways of bringing community into her life and this year is hosting a foreign exchange student from Germany.

Redefinition of Masculinity

Ned Fielden
T8
Age at SCI: 34
Date of SCI: July 22, 1989
San Francisco, California

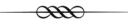

*I*t was a beastly hot Saturday afternoon in July 1989, the first day of my two-week summer vacation. I had just moved with my wife and two young kids from San Francisco to Healdsburg, a beautiful, small winery town in Sonoma County, a couple of hours to the north. At around 6 p.m., after an hour spent pushing the hand-mower around the front yard in the hundred degree heat had left me dripping with sweat, I mounted my bike to head down to the Russian River a half mile away for a cleansing plunge. It was the last proper swim I would ever have.

Cooled and feeling much better about life, I cycled back across the narrow bridge over the river. My thoughts drifted to the beauty of the rural surroundings on this first day of vacation from my job as an auto mechanic. Unknown to and unseen by me, a local yutz in a pickup truck came barreling along the road behind me, clipping the door of a parked car. Not one to stop for some petty property damage, in his hurry to get away he drove his truck bumper into my bike, tossing my body into the steel truss structure of the bridge. Hit and run.

It felt like someone had whacked me in the back with a two-ton two-by-four. As I recovered consciousness, I found myself upended, my legs thrown into the steel bridgework above me. My first sensation was the pounding pain in the middle of my back, the second the eerie observation that while my legs were rivulets of blood, I could feel no pain from them at all.

A couple of days later, after they had carted me off to a local hospital while my HMO tried to figure out what to do with me, officially a T8 paraplegic, I had a conversation with a very sweet but cautious rehab doctor.

"Do you have any idea of the extent of your injuries?" he asked softly.

"Yes, pretty good. Flattened pelvis, punctured lung, but most of all a busted back."

"Do you know what that means?"

I had already figured this one out.

"I probably won't ever walk again." I felt oddly detached in this conversation, as if we were talking about someone else's predicament. I had grasped the essentials of the situation, but also knew instinctively that a drastically altered life was waiting for me around the corner — a life that I couldn't possibly imagine at that moment.

He seemed relieved to be dealing with someone willing to face facts. He also turned out to be the kindest and sanest of any rehab doctor I would ever meet. He treated me like an intelligent, sentient being — not an oddity or annoyance. I wish to hell I'd had a chance to work with him and not some of the other village idiots I would soon encounter, once they figured out what hospital would finally stitch me up.

It took six long, hard months to figure out a direction, and over a year to get my insurance company to pay up, as they bobbed and weaved and dodged their responsibilities — despite my having faithfully paid years of premiums. Only at knife-point ("lawyer-point," to be more accurate) did they relent, and a settlement gained me a couple of years of breathing room. But by then the marriage was over, and most of my support structure in tatters. Friends were far away and suddenly hard to reach, and all my normal coping mechanisms, such as athletics, were no longer adequate or satisfying.

The country house was emptied, and I reluctantly followed my kids when they moved with their mother back to the greater San Francisco Bay Area.

Early post-accident, I got on the phone and started talking to everyone I knew who had a potentially interesting job. An old friend had gone to library school and had the best balance in his career — did interesting work with interesting people, and didn't seem in any danger of burning out. Much to everyone's surprise Vocational Rehab agreed to pay for grad school. Because I had scored high on one of their tests, I think they saw me as a good long term risk; my ultimate salary would be higher than normal, and that meant more tax dollars back in the Treasury. I went on to earn master's degrees in history, and in library and information studies. Then I entered an historically female profession, though that wasn't a conscious factor in my choice. All this took three very long years.

Grad school and my newfound student friends were about the only personally pleasurable things that happened to me during this time. Virtually every part of my life connected to my past was painful to some degree. I could still play baseball with my five-year-old son, Gene, but pitching to him was light years different. I still had to work out the dichotomy between my old "abled" life and my new vastly different landscape.

Gradually, I got to chalk up my achievements on their own merit. New people in my life didn't deal with Ned, the old friend who could change a VW engine in half an hour. They met Ned, the quick study who happened to be in a wheelchair. My two-year-old daughter, Maggie, and I shared the pleasure of riding around town with her on my lap. She felt like royalty on her perch and squealed with pleasure when whizzing downhill at a ferocious clip.

I hadn't realized just how deeply it was possible to be unhappy. Losing use of my body and all the other trappings of civilized life accumulated over thirty-four years was enormously difficult. It was a tear-soaked, depressing, demoralizing time that expended my reserves of patience and energy. I had even wondered, one particularly hopeless night, if it was possible to become dehydrated from crying too much.

Every sign of pain in someone else was a trigger for my own. Worse, every sign of pleasure in someone else (a cyclist, a game of Frisbee, a couple walking hand-in-hand on the beach) triggered tears as well. I had never envied anyone my whole life, and now I envied an eighty-year old man who could hobble out his front door and pick up his own newspaper. Every morning it was a struggle to lift my dead legs out of bed and toss them back in the saddle for another day. But I felt I had no choice. My kids, and their need to have a father — one who didn't give up — drove me. While they wished my accident hadn't happened, Gene and Maggie were sweet, wonderful, inquisitive beings. It didn't matter whether I was in a wheelchair or not, only that I was there for them. I owe them, big time.

The dissolution of my marriage was devastating in its own right — an insult upon injury. My wife insisted over and over again that my disability had nothing to do with our troubles, but from my point of view the accident had altered everything. I had been a happy, productive person, and felt happily married up to the point of the death of half of my body.

The truth is likely somewhere in between. She felt emotionally abandoned as I coped with my own depression, and we had not done well handling the grief over the change in our sexual life. Down deep, I believe she wanted to break up, and so found increasing cause to be angry with me. The further she distanced from me, the more I clutched at her, which she then found oppressive, and the harder I clutched — a cycle familiar to many broken relationships.

The overturning of roles was also likely a large part of our troubles — I had gone from very "masculine" employment (ninety-nine percent guys) as an auto mechanic to a stay-at-home dad and student. I had lost all my "normal" guy roles (big home repairs, putting up fences, digging ditches, mowing the damn lawn). My confidence was rattled to the roots. To carry on, I was faced with a drastic redefinition of masculinity.

As my very wonderful psychotherapist noted, no accident of this magnitude can help but shred some marital fabric. We had exhausted the vital residual goodwill that needs to be built up and held in reserve for successful relationships. Looking back, I should have trusted my own self-reliance much more and had confidence in my ability to pull myself out of tough situations. At the time, that was too much to ask.

In grad school, I discovered that my sense of humor had acquired — as a result of my near-death experiences and all the other extracurricular social absurdities of wheelchair life — a devastating swiftness and acerbic tenor that others found attractive. In library school, irreverence was appealing, even to my chief victims — the faculty. I was one of two students chosen to speak at the Library School graduation at Berkeley in 1992. My words were barbed and, judging from the audience response, at least passably amusing.

During the last few months of the program I had begun to date a couple of the other students. My first date, three years post-accident and my first in fifteen years, was nerve-wracking to an unimaginable degree for the whole two hours we had lunch. She with the shining almond eyes, fetching smile and soft insight. Me with more baggage than a nineteenth century Klondike mining mule. Dating became a "whattaya got to lose?" proposition. In this case, I was so smitten that it would have taken a tank of sharks to keep me from trying to get to know her better.

The ethics of the situation seemed impossible. When and how does one begin the process of full disclosure? How do you tell someone you have a defunct marriage, two kids who stop by to stay a few days a week, and a lower body which not only doesn't walk, but doesn't do much of anything except get in the way and hurt? Luckily no one turned tail straight away.

My first job was extremely part-time — I had picked a bad time to be a new librarian in California, as a recession was in full swing. The library director at Sonoma State University had queried her own brood of librarians, and it seemed that the only librarian position that might pose problems to someone in a wheelchair was reference, since you needed to dash around the collection with a certain amount of manic energy. Naturally, I had to try it just to see if I could do it, and arranged for an internship there. I was driven and focused to an extraordinary degree and felt I had to prove to every naysayer that I not only was an adequate librarian, but superior. The internship led to part-time work, and some teaching.

I landed a job as a librarian at San Francisco State University in 1995, got tenure and a promotion in 2001, and have not looked back. Academic life has its own absurdities, but my hypothesis is that people with disabilities are unusually adept at coping with the Byzantine structure of university culture, having the experience we do with Kafka-esque bureaucracies. We don't give up easily.

Best of all, I married a wonderful fellow library school student, whom my kids took to with unflinching enthusiasm. For many months, I lived the kind of charmed life reserved only for lovers. I looked forward to the end of each day when I could make dinner for Lucy and ask her the thousand and one questions about her life that had been brewing in my brain all day. I never could have imagined, in the dark months post-accident, this progression and how nice it would be. We got married in June 1996, three years after we met and almost six years after my accident. We had figured out real fast that kids were not going to happen the easy way, and with the help of the very latest in reproductive technology (and a quarter of a year's salary) we were able to conceive and raise two more kids, who are not just the apple, but the orchard, of their father's eye. Five-year old Aaron still gets to ride on my lap on the flat and downhill (too heavy for uphill now) and my two-year old Heather goes everywhere on my lap. They are my scouts and future — long live kids everywhere!

Ned Fielden lives in Berkeley California with his wonderful wife Lucy, teenagers Maggie and Gene (when he is home from college) and youngsters Aaron and Heather. He is a reference and instructional librarian at San Francisco State University and has written on Internet Search Engines.

Capable Shogaisha

Miki Matheson
C5
Age at SCI: 19
Date of SCI: October 25, 1993
Clarence-Creek, Ontario

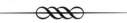

*I*n October 1993, I dreamed of becoming a physical education teacher. I loved being active. I loved playing sports, and I loved riding my mountain bike. Then everything I loved to do and hoped for seemed no longer a possibility for me.

It was a beautiful, sunny morning as I was making the one-hour bicycle ride from my house to Tokyo Gakugei University. The crosswalk light changed over to "WALK," but as I crossed a huge truck was coming through, not reducing its speed.

The driver had been asleep at the wheel, and didn't notice me until he hit me with his 18-wheeler, sending me flying almost 100 feet. He came to a stop only inches from where I had landed. Three different places of my spine were broken, injuring my spinal cord permanently.

I didn't know any of these things until after I woke up from my three-month coma. I couldn't believe this had happened to me. I didn't want to believe that it wasn't possible to recover. I didn't want to endure people calling me "Sho-ga-i-sha," an unflattering Japanese word for a disabled person that made me imagine someone who is pitiful, sad, and dependent.

When I was a child, a school for children with physical or mental disabilities was not far from our house. One day, one of our neighbors who went there was waiting for the bus, screaming crazily and shouting words I couldn't understand. I ran away, terribly scared, not knowing what to do. I asked my teacher what was wrong with him, but she didn't answer me, so I never asked anybody again. I just put it deep in my heart, sealing it with the words "too taboo to ask!" Another day, I heard some older students passing this guy saying, "Hold your breath guys, otherwise we will become fucked-up like him." These were the only ideas I had about life with a disability.

When I was told that I would never walk again, the image of that guy appeared in my mind. I suffered from intense nightmares for several days. Even though I had survived and mostly accepted my situation, my fear grew bigger every day until it drained all of my self-confidence. I was scared that I would have to deal with the attitude of those older students.

Back when I was in fourth grade, one of my best friends and I were talking about our future life. "One day, a lovely guy will find me," I said, "and he'll ask me to marry, then ..."

She started crying. I didn't know what was going on until she confessed her biggest secret — the guy screaming at the bus stop was her big brother. I had visited her house often, but never knew he was there. She told me that most people with disabilities were hidden in their homes, and the family and relatives were supposed to be ashamed of them. She cried because she had been told that, with a disabled person in her family, she would never have a chance to marry.

As I remembered my friend's tears, I became worried for my three sisters, and — of course — for myself. It seemed that the sleeping truck driver changed not only my body, but also my family's potential future. I wished I could escape from the situation I was in. I didn't yet have enough mental strength to face the harsh reality. If I had caused the accident through my own wrong actions, like drinking and driving, I could have blamed it on myself. But I hadn't done anything wrong that morning. Why had this happened to me?

I was happy to see my friends and family when they visited me in the hospital. When they left, I always wondered if they saw me as a disabled person or not. Some people asked me how I could smile even though I had to live with a wheelchair for the rest of my life. Did they have sympathy? Did they come to see me out of curiosity? Sometimes I thought that I would never go out with my wheelchair so that people would never know I was paralyzed.

Dr. Keiichi Shibasaki at National Murayama Hospital changed my weird way of thinking. I was still strapped on the bed, my face swollen, missing front teeth, immobilized by skull traction, and attached to a respirator. I was not a person — I was like a part of the machines in the room. Nobody would think I would ever play sports again, but he did. He looked at my tanned skin and simply asked me if I would like to go for swim. I loved swimming. I would do anything to go swimming!

But I couldn't say yes instantly. I was not sure I would be able to swim like before. I was not sure that I was ready to show my paralyzed body to others. He must have been reading my mind when he casually asked me, "How can you expect others to see your potential if you don't see it in yourself?"

That changed something inside me. I was so relieved to know that there was a person who could see my potential, not my disadvantage. That was the moment I came back to being my true "Miki." No longer was I "a girl trapped in a wheelchair to be pitied." He told me about many opportunities for people with spinal cord injuries. Two things caught my ears and perked them up. I could drive a car, and also participate in sports.

I had devoted myself to sports my whole life, but I didn't know that there was an Olympics for disabled athletes called the Paralympics. Through the rehab program, I practiced for wheelchair racing and sometimes beat men who had the same level as my injury, which made me smile secretly. I realized that I was still me. I was still alive! When I was training, I didn't care what part of my body was disabled and weak; I just focused on what I could do to be better, faster, or stronger. I realized my attitude was the biggest barrier I had to overcome.

One day, Dr. Shibasaki took me out of the hospital to go for a swim. In Japan, each district is supposed to have an accessible sports facility exclusively for people with disabilities. They have features like air bubbles in the pool to tell blind swimmers where the wall is, Braille on the floor, and flashing signals to catch deaf people's attention. He took me to the one in Tokyo, not far from the hospital and my house. I had a chance to see people living a "real" life using a wheelchair. I met a couple of wheelchair athletes there and was so amazed by the size of their arms. I realized that I was not watching their disability. I just couldn't keep my eyes away from their capabilities. I wanted to be just like them, not ordinary wheelchair users but really cool wheelchair athletes. I started thinking that I did not mind being called "shogaisha," so long as people think I am a "capable-shogaisha."

On that same day, I was told that I could continue my university course to be a physical education teacher. I was afraid of being rejected from the course or being told I should change from teaching. I knew that many patients around my age were told to quit school or were forced to take satellite courses, often just because of the lack of accessibility. Although most of the buildings in my university are really old, without wheelchair access, as long as I was given the chance to try, I was ready to face the difficulties.

I know people in wheelchairs tend to be the center of public attention, and it used to bother me. But, once I set the goal to finish my degree and get my teacher's license, I didn't care what people said or thought they saw any longer.

I was released from the hospital after almost one year. I was also lucky to get my driver's license as a part of my rehab program.

One spring weekend, I heard shocking news on the radio while I was driving. My hero, Superman — Christopher Reeve — had broken his neck during a riding competition. One newspaper headline read, "Superman needs help!" Superman was the man who helped others, not the one to be helped. This made me think that it may not be such a bad thing to ask for help. I had a lot of friends there for me, and I realized that my pride could keep me away from the people I love most and the experiences I could have. So I went to a coffee shop on the third floor of a building with no elevator and let my friends help me. I ordered my favorite cheesecake. It was delicious beyond description, and it encouraged me to expand my life and extend my limits.

There were two different people inside me; one was the person knowing life only before my accident, the other was born just after the accident. These two were struggling through the new circumstance of my life, not knowing what to do. I knew that I had to fully digest my disability before the person inside me — the one born just after my accident — could engage the world without any fear or expectations.

Once I went back home and started participating in sporting events, these two people inside me started to understand each other. As I won more races, my confidence came back, getting stronger as I posted records. Through sports, I learned what I can do and what I cannot do, and to just focus on my capabilities.

After a couple of years, I graduated from Tokyo Gakugei University with my teacher's license for physical education. Just a couple of days before my graduation ceremony, I become a three-time gold medalist at the Nagano Paralympic Games for Ice Sledge Racing (the Paralympic equivalent to speed skating). I also set one World Record! These things proved to me that having a disability doesn't really matter. What does matter is heart.

The athletes from all over the world amazed me every day. A blind alpine skier speeding down a steep run, just listening and using his guide's voice. A cross-country skier without arms overcoming a bumpy, curvy course. A smaller sledge hockey player who hit a huge player so hard he gave the huge guy a concussion. Fearless determination and power. They all had some kind of disability, but they had something totally special as well. Disability does not dictate quality of life. The way I see myself and how I live with my disability determines my quality of my life.

The Paralympic Games were one of the most exciting and proud times of my life. The organizing committee for the 1998 winter Paralympics produced a series of posters, and they chose me as the poster girl for my sport — with "JOY" as the inspiration word. During the games, a lot of athletes asked me, "Are you the Joy girl?" and many of them told me that

I had a great smile.

When I think back to when I was first injured, I remember my despair, and how I had regretted the loss of all of life's possibilities. Today, I truly feel it was not so bad to go through. Some strangers have called my friends my "attendants." Some people baby talked to me, as though they thought I had a mental disability as well. I don't care anymore about those people who can only see part of me. I have gained power, strength, and a different point of view that I didn't have before my accident.

The biggest bonus is that I found my partner for life, the person who loved my smile the most. Shawn and I met during the Paralympics. He has been competing for Canada as a sledge hockey player since 1991. We were married in November 2001, in Japan. The whole National Canadian Sledge Hockey Team was there for us. My life with a spinal cord injury is filled with love and smiles.

Miki Matheson lives in Clarence-Creek, Ontario. She is a freelance journalist for a Japanese newspaper and various magazines, and a speaker on accessibility and disability awareness in Japan. She is the proud parent of a beautiful Bernese Mountain dog, Hana, and is dreaming of being the next triathlete champion of "Iron-Women."

New Dreams

Jim Langevin
C6-7
Age at SCI: 16
Date of SCI: August 22, 1980
Warwick, Rhode Island

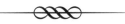

*G*rowing up in Rhode Island, I always liked structure and the idea of being a part of something larger than myself. Law enforcement had a particular appeal to me. The idea of public service and protecting my community always made sense. As a kid, it was my dream to put on a blue uniform and chase down the bad guys. I wanted more than anything else to be a police officer or maybe even an FBI agent. When I was thirteen (1977), I began to participate in a Boy Scout Explorer/Police Cadet program in my hometown of Warwick. The program gave young people the opportunity to explore a possible career in law enforcement, by working with police both on the road and in the police station. Through this program, my interest grew stronger, and I felt well on my way to an honorable career.

At sixteen, my lifelong dream ended one afternoon in the police locker room. Two police officers were looking at a new gun, which they did not realize was loaded. The gun accidentally fired, and the bullet went through my neck, cutting my spinal cord at C6-7.

Hours later, after being in and out of consciousness, I woke up in the emergency room, heavily medicated and unaware of the extent of my injuries. I was later transferred to University Hospital in Boston for longer-term care. Although my doctors and family had decided not to tell me the severity of my injury right away, I soon began to ask questions of everyone who walked into my room. As I put the pieces together, a nurse explained that I had a spinal cord injury and would not be able to walk.

While I understood what people were telling me, subconsciously I believed that I would be fine because I had been hospitalized years before when I was sick, and had gotten better. I just couldn't believe that this had happened. As each day passed, it became clear that recovery was unlikely anytime soon.

Emotionally, it was overwhelming. I cried many nights, and felt sad and a sense of emptiness. The emotional wounds were deep. It was very frustrating to have to re-learn how to do things. Learning to breathe was very difficult — especially since I had to do it on my back, in traction, with those awful tongs attached to my head.

My parents and other members of my family visited me every day for the five months that I was hospitalized. My parents never let on about the extent of their grief. Only later did I learn that they were "basket cases" emotionally and would cry and console one another at home. They and my brothers were very supportive just by being there. Their loving support meant a great deal. My baby sister Joanne visited too, and our time with her provided a joyful escape. Although she was only three months old, she helped our family in our darkest moments just by being a cute baby who needed attention and love. She helped us learn to smile again. I also had a lot of support from my friends, people at the police department, and others in the community.

Letting go of my dream of becoming a police officer was a slow and painful process. It was especially difficult for me to talk with my good friend who was also in the cadet program because he was able to proceed with his plans. Looking back, it was like going through a death and being slowly reborn into a new life. My strong religious faith helped me reach inside myself to find strength and courage. My faith in God sustained me and grew stronger as I recognized that He would provide me with all I needed to get through these difficult times. I believe that God has a plan for all of us. I also believe that God sends specific people into each of our lives when we need them, and these people enable us to learn, grow, and succeed.

I finally returned home in the middle of my sophomore year. I wanted to finish high school and graduate with my class. But I was very nervous about going back because I had a heavy load of schoolwork and would need to get around in my wheelchair. Brother John Beilen, my principal at Bishop Hendricken High School, had visited me several times in the hospital and was great when I returned to school. Initially, I was tutored in Brother Beilen's office so that I could catch up, feel more confident, and get re-acclimated to the school environment. Gradually, I rejoined my classmates.

As I returned to high school rituals, such as writing term papers, there were obstacles. The only way I could type my papers was to weave a pen through my fingers and peck out the words, one letter at a time. This certainly wasn't the most efficient way to do a term paper, so I begged my mother, a former secretary, to type them for me. I was frustrated and very angry when she insisted that I could do it on my own. Having very little choice, I typed every single one of those papers myself, using an old electric typewriter.

Mom also pushed me to get out and do things, while Dad reined her in when she pushed too hard. Mom and Dad complemented each other — together they provided for me, let me do things at my own pace, and encouraged me to be independent.

I was cautious about being out in the community, and I didn't like people staring at me. I decided for myself when I would go out. Since I was already a coin collector, I began by going to coin shows again with my brothers and friends.

Time and time again, my family, friends, and community came through for me. When my parents found out that my friend and fellow cadet, Cathy, was having some problems at home, they invited her to stay with us and be part of our family. Cathy continues to be a good friend —

to this day. My parents also cared for a number of foster children over the years, and continued to do so after my accident. The nature of my family, to be so engaged in society, was a constant reminder that I was part of an extended, caring community — at a time when it would have been easy to feel isolated.

During this time, I was also reevaluating my future. My childhood dreams had been suddenly dashed. As I confronted new challenges, I was faced many times with the choice between sitting back and letting life pass me by or deciding to get out and live. I decided to reengage myself in my community and develop new dreams. I chose to live.

After my accident, I became a more serious student. But, I was apprehensive about college because it meant leaving the comfort and security of home. Part of me wanted to stay home and be safe in its warm cocoon. However, my parents were determined that I attend college and not hide at home. I only applied to two schools — Providence College (PC), my first choice, and Rhode Island College (RIC). I was thrilled to be accepted at PC, and began to grow excited at the prospect of beginning the life of a college student. In the summer before I was to begin, I went on a tour of the campus. Going from building to building, I grew more and more concerned and disappointed — the campus was not designed with accessibility in mind. I realized that I would not be able to go to PC.

Touring the campus of my back-up school was more reassuring. Accommodations at RIC were not perfect, but they were years ahead of their time — this was almost ten years before the Americans with Disabilities Act. RIC provided me with a quality education and the opportunity to put some of my new dreams to the test.

Because my mom worked for the City of Warwick and had involved my brothers and me on political campaigns, I had some interest in politics and government. I decided to run for freshman class representative in the student government. Winning that election was a defining moment for me, and my subsequent service in student government reinforced my interest in politics. The RIC student government was a parliamentary system and, over the next few years, my colleagues elected me vice president and then president of the student body. However, I still wasn't thinking of politics as a career.

In my junior year, remembering all that my community had done for me and wanting to give something back, I ran successfully for a position as a delegate to Rhode Island's Constitutional Convention, which redrafted the state's constitution. I was getting more and more interested in politics and public service, finding that I enjoyed making a difference in my community. In my senior year, I decided to run for the Rhode Island General Assembly. I didn't worry much about how I would manage to campaign or serve if elected. Instead, I just jumped in and felt confident that everything would work out fine. I've always had a can-do attitude.

Getting elected meant campaigning door-to-door and going to rallies in the district I had lived in all my life. For our door-to-door campaigning, my friends rang doorbells on each side of a street, told people I was on the street, and invited people to come out and meet me. Although many people knew me and/or knew about my accident, I didn't know how people would react to me as a candidate. I knew that people needed to see me working hard to get elected. As I was campaigning, it became clear that people who didn't know me had a natural curiosity about my disability, and that became a minor distraction from my message. As my career progressed, I learned to address the issue up front in speeches, so that we could move on.

While serving in the state legislature, I received my bachelor's degree in political science and was accepted to a master's program at the Kennedy School of Government at Harvard University. Commuting an hour and fifteen minutes each way, I finished in May 1994, and ran for and won the office of Secretary of State in November. I was reelected in 1998. In 2000, I won a seat in the United States House of Representatives, and have been honored to represent my home state in Washington, D.C., ever since.

I am determined not to let life pass me by. In the weeks, months, and even years after my accident, I had to let go of my old dreams and develop the patience and perspective that guide me today. I grew to understand what Hemingway meant when he said, "The world breaks everyone, and afterward many are strong at the broken places." The twenty-three years I have lived since the accident have been full of life and passion, and many of my new dreams of public service have been fulfilled.

These years have also seen major changes for people with disabilities in America. It is easier for me to shop and go to the movies than it was in the 1980s, and Providence College is now an accessible campus — I've been back from time to time to lecture. People with disabilities today, myself included, benefit tremendously from the ADA and other laws that have leveled the playing field. The ADA has resulted in changes that go far beyond physical structures like ramps and Braille signs. By establishing that we have equal rights, this law changed the way society perceives us — we have the right to participate in and contribute to society. This was made possible by determined advocates who came before us — pioneers, who in the face of great adversity, cracked open the doors. I believe that it is up to each of us to continue to open and go through those doors and discover our own potential. I view this as an obligation, and I am proud to give back to my community in honor of those who came before me.

As a member of Congress, I go back and forth to Washington each week even though I'm a homebody kind of person. Every day, I get up at 5 or 6 a.m. to get ready for work with the assistance of my home health aide. It takes me three hours — I'm one of the lucky ones because I have access to quality care. My busy and active life keeps me from dwelling on the negative. I know there will always be moments from time to time when I feel down, but don't we all? However, over time, these moments have become fewer and farther apart.

I'm glad that I found the courage to work toward my new dreams. I plan to keep on dreaming.

Jim Langevin lives in Warwick, Rhode Island. He represents the people of the Second Congressional District of Rhode Island as a Member of the United States House of Representatives in Washington, DC. He travels back and forth between Rhode Island and Washington weekly, and enjoys spending time with his family and friends.

Lucky Man

Victor Cerda
C3
Age at SCI: 20
Date of SCI: May 1, 1986
Tyler, Texas

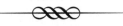

Seventeen years ago, May 1, 1986, five days before my twenty-first birthday, I was involved in an unusual vehicular accident when my truck collided with a full-sized horse. That's how I became a C3 quad. My lovely wife, Sherry, and I had been married only fifteen months. Sherry and I did our rehabilitation in Houston at The Institute for Rehabilitation and Research (T.I.R.R.). I include Sherry because she was there with me every step of the way.

Immediately after my injury, we realized our lives would change, but we didn't know just how. Before getting admitted to the rehab center, we had our sights set on going home. It didn't take long for us to realize that we were in no shape to go home and start our new lives. We had no prior training on how to take care of a quad, did not own a wheelchair, and had no idea where to buy medical supplies. And, we had no knowledge about how to manage my personal needs such as my bowels and bladder.

After conquering the smaller tasks of our disability like learning how to use a mouth stick and educating ourselves on how to manage my fluids, we soon realized that we had larger responsibilities and challenges to overcome. Learning how to operate and maintain a power wheelchair and making our house accessible were two major challenges. Getting re-educated for possible employment was another. When I didn't regain function in my extremities and it became obvious that I was not going to regain use of my legs, we knew our lives were going to be very different. Realizing this and coming to terms with it was a big part of the rehabilitation process.

People react to such life changing tragedies in different ways. Some people might go into a deep depression and others may slip into denial. As far as we were concerned, Sherry and I knew that we could either laugh about it or cry about it. The love that we continued to have for one another helped us come to this conclusion. We went through this together and were able to discuss it with one another. We quickly learned that it is a lot easier, and more fun, to laugh than it is to cry about such changes.

We did not have a van with a wheelchair lift. As a result, Sherry had to transfer me in and out of a regular passenger car. She might as well have been picking me up off of the ground. My therapist at the rehab center trained us on how to do transfers. We did this while my tracheotomy was still in my throat. It was difficult in the beginning, but the bottom line is that we had no choice. We did what we had to do. I suppose that as Texans, we knew it was a matter of "taking the bull by the horns." Nowadays, Sherry sometimes picks me up and carries me from room to room. Fortunately, I weigh only one hundred and twenty-three pounds.

I didn't break down and cry until several months post injury when I saw Sherry in the reflection of a mirror pushing me down the hall in what seemed like a two-ton manual wheelchair. I'll never forget it. We had just completed our first three months in rehabilitation and were home on a weekend pass. After seeing us in the mirror, my first thought was, "Wow, we are much too young for this type of life." Then I thought, "How could such a loving and kind woman have something like this happen to her?" Prior to seeing our reflection in the mirror, I don't think I had ever really felt disabled. This was not a time when we were laughing. I felt as though I had failed our marriage and let down my wife.

A lot of hugs — and time — got us through this difficult experience.

I can recall several times at T.I.R.R when I thought about how our lives would be different and wondered how we would cope with the challenges to come. I remember lying in a big room with other patients doing physical therapy when the physical therapist told me that I would need to start each day with a series of exercises. How would I do that? I also remember sitting in occupational therapy typing letters to our friends and family members with a device called a mouthstick. The therapist had placed it in my mouth and I knew exactly what to do with it. I was "a natural." I was soon typing twenty words a minute. Since then, I've always told Sherry that I guess I was born to be a quad. Using the mouthstick continues to be a daily part of my life and has contributed to my independence. From that experience, I have learned to never underestimate my inner strength.

I had lots of time to think — and worry — about our new circumstances. But, I knew that we were not alone and that Sherry and I would work through this together. I thank God for blessing me with a loving and caring wife who was with me every day during the rehabilitation process and who continues to be by my side today. We knew and continue to realize that our God would not give us something that we could not handle. Just as Sherry was there for me, her parents and siblings as well as my extended family were also there for us. I truly believe that without God's blessings and without our family members' love, support, and prayers, we could not have made it through those difficult times.

We had been very concerned about how we were going to make a living and pay our bills. After several months in rehab, I really wanted to go back to work. I had enjoyed working with my hands manufacturing computers. But, immediately after my injury, I knew that I would be unable to continue. Five months after my injury, I visited my employer. In addition to realizing that it was time to start something new, I really appreciated that my co-workers were concerned about our well-being. It was time to go back to the classroom for retraining.

I had graduated from high school with no aspirations of going to college. During my high school days, I believed I was not suited for college. I thought I lacked the patience to sit in a classroom — until someone at the rehab center told me that I was not college material. I wanted to prove him wrong. Although I was supposedly "not college material," I registered for my first semester anyway. I went to college with an aide and began using my brain again. I ended up attending college for several years. The most important lesson I learned was that I could function on my own for several hours without my Sherry. Four years ago, we decided to put college off and do some traveling around this beautiful country of ours. Because of the benefits that my former employer has blessed us with, we are able to support ourselves and take the occasional trips that we enjoy very much.

During the first several years, we had our moments as we learned how to work together and listen to each other. Today, we can laugh at our memories of the learning process. Our first solo transfer at home from the car to my manual chair was on a very hot day, at least ninety degrees. Sherry had me in her arms and I was trying to instruct her on how to complete the transfer safely. I told her to go one way; she wanted to go another. After a few well-chosen words at one another, we got through it. We also learned about getting through shaving even though when we first started I was annoyed that she wasn't using enough shaving cream and told her to use the entire can. At the same time, I was patient and told Sherry that I appreciated her efforts. Because I didn't want to do weight shifts in my chair to prevent pressure sores as often as Sherry thought I should, she has gently reminded me how important it is with great results — no sores.

We have also been able to laugh together about "mistakes." Once, Sherry forgot to strap down the front of manual chair in the van and I landed on my back when she stopped at the first red light. When she asked if she could take my picture while I was face up, I laughed and agreed. We were also able to laugh when my power chair was broken and she left me in the back yard in my manual chair — and forgot where she had put me!

After what seemed like a long rehabilitation process, we moved to Beaumont, Texas. After living in Beaumont for four years, we relocated to beautiful East Texas. We feel that Tyler, where we currently live, is our own little corner of the world.

A lot of people have asked me about "the cure," and whether I would consider another surgery. I would consider it — if it were a hundred percent guaranteed. But, few things in life are. For now, we are both very happy.

Mark Chesnutt, a country music singer, sings a song entitled "Lucky Man." A lot of my feelings and thoughts about my life are in the lyrics.

I've got things to be down about,
But in spite of it all, honey, ain't no doubt,
I'm livin' the life of a lucky man.

I could be down about losing the use of my extremities; yet, I'm lucky to have Sherry by my side.

So many things to talk about
That never do come true;
Oh, heaven knows,
I wish they could for you.

I wish I could walk again just so I could dance with Sherry.

Believe me, I know you should be tempted to go;
Oh, that would be the easy thing to do.
So many just give up and walk away.
In spite of it all, you're strong enough to stay.
Oh, I'm livin' the life of a lucky man.

This last one is my favorite part of the song because it really describes Sherry.

God has blessed Sherry with the strength and patience to endure some difficult circumstances in our marriage. For that I am thankful, and truly "livin' the life of a lucky man."

If I have learned one thing from this new life, it is that Sherry did not marry me because I was able-bodied. We have learned how to take the bitter with the sweet and roll on. We helped each other learn through patience, love, and communication — and learning from our mistakes. It seems that learning how to deal with life's challenges is something that has come naturally to us. We have always been problem solvers. Overcoming the little challenges in life prepared us for the even larger obstacles. There are tough times in life. Not every building has been accessible, and there are potholes in every road. We hope to see you on the road as we travel.

Victor Cerda lives in Tyler, Texas, with Sherry, his wife of eighteen years. Vic keeps busy working on his computer, reading, painting, and traveling with Sherry.

Wife, Mother, Me

Faye Pruitt
T8
Age at SCI: 20
Date of SCI: August 24, 1968
Newberg, Oregon

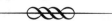

At twenty, I had finished my sophomore year in college, was preparing to teach elementary music, and was engaged to a boy I loved very much. My health was good — I was athletic and enjoyed sports.

In August 1968, after becoming engaged to Bill Pruitt, we were driving to a camp in Estacada, Oregon, where we were leading music. Our car did not have seat belts. It was dark, raining, and we were in a hurry. We didn't make it around the curve. We ended up in a ravine and hit a tree. Bill was thrown out, hit a tree, broke his collarbone, and was bruised up. I stayed in the car; my back was broken at the T8 level, and I was paralyzed from the rib cage down.

I spent three months in Providence Hospital in Portland, six weeks of those on a Stryker turning frame. Bill spent most of each day with me while his collarbone was healing. I couldn't talk much at first, but just having him there was such a comfort. He felt guilty and wished he had been more careful. I told him that I still loved him, and my father assured him that we didn't blame him. That relieved him of a lot of feelings of guilt.

I couldn't believe that Bill would still find me attractive. I was not glamorous lying on the Stryker turning frame, with IVs and tubes attached to my body, disheveled hair, scrapes and bruises all over, and nurses, doctors and therapists doing everything for me. But, he told me he still loved me and planned on sticking around — that was a miracle! It showed me the depth of his love and that it wasn't just based on physical attraction or our ability to have fun together. I was so grateful.

I didn't face the reality of my disability in the hospital. When the head of the physical therapy department showed me pictures of people walking with leg braces and crutches and using wheelchairs, I brushed it all aside by making jokes. I didn't want to deal with it as a possible part of my future. I had been healthy and athletic. Leg braces, crutches, and wheelchairs didn't belong in my image of who I was. I was told that whatever return of function I would have would come within six months. We were in a "wait and see" mode.

After three months, I was transferred to the Rehabilitation Institute of Oregon. Over two months as an inpatient, and six weeks as an outpatient, I came to grips with the finality of my disability. As time passed, I had no return of function. I remember a growing awareness that my paralysis wasn't going away. The doctors and therapists didn't give me any false hopes. They worked at preparing me to live life from a wheelchair.

All my time and energy went into learning the things I needed to know to take care of myself as a paraplegic. It was overwhelming. I was exhausted physically, because I was doing everything with just my arm and chest muscles. The first time I dressed myself, including putting on my leg braces, it took two hours. At the end of that time, I was ready for a nap, but I had hours of therapy ahead.

I was surrounded by people who were also learning to cope with lifelong disabilities. They reminded me of who I was — but didn't want to be. Even though I knew I looked just like all the others in wheelchairs, I really didn't view myself like that.

Because I couldn't hide from reality anymore, I experienced much more depression. I don't remember ever talking about this with doctors. I did have a very open relationship with my physical therapist and confided in her sometimes.

It felt like all the joy of life was gone forever. My view of people with disabilities was that they were very dependent on others for everything. I couldn't imagine functioning as a wife, working person, or mother (if I could have children) — a normal person — when all my time and energy went in to the daily routine of maintaining hygiene, dressing myself, doing physical therapy, etc.

My faith in God, as well as the support of people who loved me and prayed for me, carried me during this time. I focused on God's Biblical promises: God was going to bring good out of this difficult situation; He would give me strength to bear it; and I did have hope for a future. I believed God didn't lie, so these promises were true whether I felt them or not.

I wanted to be independent again. My whole day was spent learning things I had learned as a small child, such as toilet training and dressing, and how to keep healthy as a paraplegic. While I felt like giving up many times, in my heart, I didn't want to. Over and over, I repeated to myself (silently), "I won't give up, I won't give up," and I prayed that God would help me.

During rehab, I met a young woman who had polio as a child and had been using a wheelchair many years. She was married and the mother of three. She took care of her home and children, shopped, drove, and seemed very normal. This first glimpse at the possible gave me great hope that I wouldn't just be a burden to Bill — I could actually be a good wife.

My first year of living with a disability was very hard. I was tired physically, and it took much emotional energy to go out into the "real world" and be with "real people," knowing that I might be a spectacle if my legs went into spasms or something embarrassing happened. After that first year, life gradually began to take on some semblance of normalcy. I chose not to continue preparing to teach music. Instead, Vocational Rehabilitation paid my way through business college. Then, I was hired as a secretary at George Fox University in Newberg, Oregon, where Bill continued his education.

We were married eighteen months after our accident. For the next three years, I worked at the university while Bill finished his degree. I was often exhausted, but it was also a good time for me. Knowing I could work and help support us did so much for my self-esteem. I also learned to drive again.

I worked until I was six months pregnant with Michelle. Although I had a normal pregnancy, I had to convince my doctor not to do a C-section. I gave him information, given to me by my therapist at RIO, showing it was possible for a paraplegic to have a normal birth. He agreed to let me try. Shelly was three weeks overdue — and I had a month of false labor — but she was born vaginally, although the doctor did use forceps. Our son, Jeremy, was born three and a half years later. This time we took the child birth classes. Jeremy was a natural birth with Bill in the delivery room. My labor pains were very intense, and caused double vision and headaches for several days after his birth — just as I had read was normal for a mother with spinal cord injury.

Because I grew up in a large family with younger sisters that I helped care for, being a mother wasn't as overwhelming for me as it might have been. It was tiring, and my back was sore most of the time from picking up and holding my babies with just my arms and chest muscles. But, I loved my babies and the feeling of being so needed.

I nursed both of my children for a year. I taught them to hang onto my armrests at five months of age by working with them over and over, putting their hands on the armrests and telling them to hang on. After about a week, they learned to hang on so I could roll with them sitting on my lap without holding onto them. After my children learned to walk, I taught them to hang onto my armrests and walk beside me whenever we went someplace. They continued this habit all through their growing-up years.

I loved being a mother; I'm so glad I had the privilege. Like most mothers, I was very tired during their preschool years. Just the same, it's the best thing I've ever done.

Since Bill was on the pastoral staff in churches in the area of music and support ministries, we had been giving to people all the time, as well as to our children at home. Our own needs and our relationship were secondary to the needs of others. In our forties, this caught up with us. The emotional needs that we had not recognized or dealt with earlier came to the forefront as our children were growing up and leaving the nest.

While I was not physically dependent on Bill for personal care, and I had maintained our household and cared for our children, I believe I was emotionally dependent on him for encouragement when I was down — and he was good at giving it. I think my disability gave Bill more of a sense of responsibility for me.

I am glad Bill is an optimist. But I believe he didn't really grieve the losses that our accident caused him. It's good to focus on the positives in life, but Bill did this to the exclusion of admitting that there really were losses for him in marrying a woman with a disability. When we married, we were young and very much in love. We did not have the wisdom or maturity that we have today and didn't recognize or deal with some of the feelings that our accident had caused.

We had a few shaky years in our marriage. We left the ministry and got counseling to help us deal with the pain we were both feeling. I learned to be more emotionally independent of Bill and made the decision to go back to work, even though I knew it would result in me being more tired. It was a transition time for me. My whole self-concept had been tied up in being a wife, mother, and a minister's wife. I had to learn who I really was, apart from those roles. And I had to learn professional skills in order to go back to work. I did not know computers until then. I went to work for Newberg Friends Church as a receptionist and publications secretary for thirty hours a week.

Bill was able to face pain and loss about our accident that he had not faced when he was younger, and to grieve the losses and accept them.

We came out the other side of those years better people, more realistic about our personal strengths and weaknesses, and thankful that we didn't throw in the towel on our relationship just because things were tough. Our marriage is stronger today, having gone through those painful years.

We have adjusted to my disability. If we had a choice we would choose for me not to be disabled. But we don't have that choice, and we both believe in accepting what we cannot change, making the best of it, and depending on God to give us the strength to do it.

Faye Pruitt lives in Newberg, Oregon, has been married thirty-four years, has two grown children, and works as a secretary/receptionist. As a hobby, she does ventriloquism and chalk art for children's groups (and sometimes adults). She and her husband also enjoy singing together.

Life After a Run at the River

Chuck Stebbins
C6-7
Age at SCI: 26
Date of SCI: July 22, 1982
Fargo, North Dakota

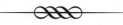

I couldn't move anything, but it didn't hurt. It was an incredibly warm feeling that I remember most, as I floated buck naked in a swimming hole in the Heart River with my neck broken at C6-7. Then some sandy-haired kid poked through the crowd of paramedics to tell me if I had faith I could walk out of there. He was gone as quickly as he popped in. How he knew I couldn't walk remains a mystery. I can't explain it rationally. That convinced me that the eighty or so odd years we spend here is not the end. There is more.

I later read Dr. Raymond Moody's book *Life After Life* and learned that a very warm feeling is one of the common things people describe in their near death experiences. That boy haunts me to this day on matters of faith. A guardian angel? Maybe.

After the third beer, I'd decided to dive off a small cliff. It was after work on a hot summer weekday, with my friend from work and his girlfriend who, sadly, wasn't interested in joining us for a little skinny dip. I had checked the depth and thought that ten feet would be plenty. So I climbed up the cliff, stepped back five feet or so, and took off. I remember hitting the water, my arms and legs not responding, running out of air and sucking in water. The next thing I know I'm lying face up in the water.

It was the summer of 1982 in Mandan, North Dakota, and I would turn twenty-seven in October. I had a wife of five years and a five-month-old son. Before breaking my neck I hadn't spent more than two or three days in a hospital. This stay was going to last three months. It sucked beyond anything I could have imagined. Needles everywhere, people wearing the same clothes, lights on all the time, a metal halo contraption fastened to my head with stainless steel screws, and some kind of tube stuck in my throat. When they told me I was a C6-7 complete quadriplegic, I didn't have a clue, nor did I care, what that meant.

All I wanted was the metal off my head and the damnable tube out of my throat. Those three months were made up of strange walking dreams, hallucinations, one nasty nurse, a stupid social worker, and non-stop needles. The drugs took the edge off the experience and made it go away for a while. Demerol. Good stuff.

Getting to rehab at Craig in Denver was a joy. It was definitely a step up from the hospital where everything was too structured, too white, too clinical, too goddamn sterile looking. The bottom line — I was not in control of anything, everyone else was. I honestly thought the guy at rehab who turned out to be my doctor was some kind of maintenance man.

At Craig, I thought I would meet the doctor in some closed setting with his nurse, all of them wearing white coats, but it didn't happen. I was beginning to feel some control here. I started meeting people my own age and younger. Somehow, that helped me see the bigger picture, helped me get beyond "Why me?" The sense of loneliness lifted a bit.

The people who were working with me were very good at this rehab thing and had the right attitude. Most of the staff were women, so it was very easy to motivate me, particularly my physical therapist and a blonde lady with a killer body who worked as an aide. (That's a hint into why I'm no longer married.) The staff treated me with respect. Not as a patient, but as a person.

My wife, Donna, came every day while I was in the hospital with our son, Jesse, but she and Jesse could only make three trips out to rehab. It was hard, but it was how it had to be. I don't believe I would have made it out of the hospital and into rehab with the attitude I did if it hadn't been for Donna and my family. Jesse, of course, was a hit with the ladies with his fuzzed out hair like he'd stuck his finger in an outlet.

I thought about how was I going to be a father to my son now. Being a new father is tough enough without a disability. Being one from a wheelchair scared the hell out of me. I would never be able wrestle or shoot baskets with him, pick him up when he's crying or just hold him. I had a son to raise, and as much bullshit as I had to deal with, it would be selfish of me — and unfair to him — to deprive him of a father. It never occurred to me that there was a whole world of cerebral stuff I hadn't even begun to explore.

As I went through rehab, I met people with higher-level injuries rolling around in sip and puffs and people with lower injuries popping wheelies and climbing curbs. I was in the middle. It felt both good and bad: I was frustrated that I didn't have as much as the T12 para, delighted that I had more than the C3-4 quad.

I learned how to transfer my dead weight around, no simple task believe me. Suddenly, every simple daily task turned into a major problem, which eventually turned into a major accomplishment. Peeing through a tube in my belly and learning how to manage a bowel program — two of the most difficult things to deal with — turned out to be no big deal. I trained my system to take a dump every third day and kept the help to a minimum.

Donna threw a nice homecoming with a few close friends when I got back from rehab. She is now my former wife (I hate the "ex" part). I believe that a big reason the relationship fell apart was because I made her my caregiver. Things became more of a chore. I think Donna felt like she couldn't go do the things she liked to do. I should have seen it and taken her away from everything to do with my care. There was more to it, but I believe my disability provided a way out, a reason not to deal with our relationship. So it just dissolved.

My marriage lasted five years after my injury. The disability took a back seat to a big ass heartache and oncoming depression. It took about three years before things stopped hurting so bad. I give Donna a boatload of credit, though. If it were not for her in those very difficult years after my injury, I would not be anywhere near where I am today. The irony is that the divorce actually helped me in more ways than it hurt. It brought me closer to the gimp's holy grail: independence.

Independence is everything to me. With the exception of taking a shit and getting in and out of the shower, I do pretty much everything else on my own. The first time I got my dead ass dressed and out of bed took me damn near two hours. When I finished my pants were twisted to the point of cutting off vital blood flow, but I was up and I was in my chair. I looked like hell, but it felt great!

When I first got home, I decided to quit taking the medications they had me on for spasticity and for my bladder. It wasn't a good idea. I was miserable for about a year. I didn't know what was wrong, and I was not talking to the right people to try and figure it out. So I stayed miserable. I got to like it after awhile. It was better than going to another hospital where you were one step away from being admitted, then stuck with needles at 6 a.m. by some freakin' vampire.

At the time, I had one of those dinosauric wheelchairs with the quad pegs and the hill climbers so you wouldn't roll backwards down the ramp and break the rest of your neck. I learned to drive at rehab, an experience in itself. On the second day out, I was amazed to be driving through downtown Denver with hand controls and paralyzed from the chest down! After that, going wherever I wanted was not a problem.

Late in 1984, I heard about a guy at the University of Minnesota who did tendon transfer surgery that could help you get a grip and a pinch — if you were a good candidate. Three operations later I had a twelve-pound grip and a five-pound pinch. It increased my independence three hundred percent. Dr. James House is one step below God in my book. Healing from those operations took most of the year, and just sitting around wasn't going to cut it. "Days of Our Lives" was really starting to suck.

So I did some volunteer work with the local Center for Independent

Living, where I learned a bit about vocational rehabilitation. I figured "I be needin' some education and shit," so I got started at a local private school in the fall of 1985. Voc Rehab helped with a few things — gas, books, and paying for an attendant to help me get going in the morning. I later learned that they could have helped with a few more things, like a bigger share of the tuition. I just didn't know it was there for me. Information truly is power.

I was terrified of going to school. My worst fear was, "What if I fall out of my chair?" I came up with the brilliant idea of tying a shoestring to the handle of my briefcase so if it started to slide off the end of my knees I could pull it back. Well the concept was a good one, but I forgot that I couldn't use my stomach muscles to help with the pulling. The case started to slide off the end of my knees and fell off, pulling me right along with it. There I sat, dead in the freakin' water.

After my legs stopped shaking — and saying the "F" word a few times — I resigned myself to the fact that there was nothing at all I could do about my situation; I would need help. Two passersby put me back in my chair. Suddenly there was no anxiety. The worst thing that could have happened already had. The next four and a half years were a piece of cake.

My grades were questionable at times, but the social experience I got in school shaped and helped me even more. I found a whole new circle of friends, most of them women — a real plus — and I had something to work toward, a goal in life, which I never really had before. Breaking my neck had actually given me some focus on finding some kind of direction. I didn't really know what that was going to be yet, but it was refreshing to feel that way.

Turns out there were a lot of things I could do with my son, Jesse. Once he got comfortable with my disability, he was just a kid, pissin' me off like any other parent. The problem was that I couldn't catch the little shit! He knew that too. Trying to reason with this six-year-old was a complete waste of time! But he made it through adolescence with a clean record, so by all indications we did the right things.

I look back on the past twenty-one years with mixed emotion. Life sucks one day, and feels pretty good the next. I've been working now for the last twelve years, off Social Security Disability, and paying taxes just like everyone else.

Quality of life is what you make it. My quality of life is as good or better than it was before my injury. As I age, I see things changing just as everyone else sees things changing. I get slower, glasses are necessary to read, I went to a power chair after nineteen years to save energy for the next twenty, my son is still my son, and I am still his father. Life is good today.

Chuck Stebbins lives in Fargo, North Dakota. He hasn't remarried, but is taking inquires. His immediate family includes his mother Lenore, stepfather Donnie, four brothers and one sister — Bob, Randy, Rick, Tim, and Roxanne, — and a large number of extended family members. He works as a community services coordinator at the Freedom Resource Center for Independent Living, where he is involved in community organizing for legislative and systems change in the disability community..

Walking the Fine Line

Mark Edwards
T4
Age at SCI: 29
Date of SCI: January 7, 2000
Fullerton, California

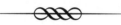

*I*t seems the only walking I will do now is on the fine line between happiness and sadness. In January of 2000, a weak blood vessel in my spinal column burst while I was sleeping. The resulting blood clot compressed my cord at the T4 level. I first felt severe chest pains and, very quickly, felt my legs start to tingle. In the time it took for me to lie down and kick one shoe off, I had lost all motor control and sensation from the chest down. Despite the loss, I was fortunate to have full use of my arms, hands, and fingers.

Twenty-nine years old and paraplegic. Not exactly how I envisioned the new year starting, or the rest of my life for that matter. I was in excellent health. I didn't smoke, rarely drank alcohol, I exercised often and kept myself in shape. Not being able to run, ride, golf, or hike makes me feel like a penniless sex addict in the Red Light District. While I did not want to distance myself from my friends, it was hard to be around people who were doing and talking about those things that I loved doing.

The first year was difficult, full of flashback memories. I'd often find myself thinking, "Last year at this time I was hiking Mt. Whitney, or Marsha and I were putting up Christmas lights." After a year had passed, I would still recall memories of better days but I would remind myself how fortunate I was to be alive to think and talk about those things. Each new day provides a blank sheet with which to create new memories. It's up to me how that day turns out. It's quite a beautiful feeling to know that.

People who suffer spinal cord injuries rarely ever walk again, but not me. I was going to be the exception; I was going to walk again, and soon. When I was in the hospital, following surgery to remove the blood clot, a physiatrist told me that I would probably be walking by my thirtieth birthday, which was two months later, March 10. Another doctor in rehab told me the same thing. What a relief. In addition, scientists were coming up with some promising results relative to nerve regeneration that could help those with spinal cord injuries to walk again. There was hope that some sort of procedure could be developed within five years, so if my body did not heal on its own, science would do it for me.

I looked at my time in rehab as a sabbatical. I was going to take four months off from work and get to work out a lot. It was close to nirvana.

Once I came home from rehab, I started researching online, looking for information about my type of injury. I learned that it does not matter how the spinal cord is injured, the only thing that matters is the severity of the injury, and my cord was compressed nearly eighty percent. Research suggests that any return of function occurs within the first three to six months after an injury. After further encounters with other people with spinal cord injuries, I realized that the "five year cure" had been talked about for the past twenty years. However, nearly four years have passed since my injury, and I have not given up hope for walking. Every day, from the moment I wake, I try to wiggle my toes or move my legs. While I still want to walk again, I want to enjoy the life I have. It's important to keep on living and making every day count.

Looking back, I can't believe how fast the time has gone. I'd like to believe it's the adage, "Time flies when you're having fun," but I'm not so sure about that. Every day presents me with a different challenge. Some days I come out ahead, and other days it seems like my path is paved with spike-strips. I've come to realize that patience, persistence, and perspective are necessities in dealing with a spinal cord injury.

I try to maintain as normal a life as possible. Outside of family, the first consideration was my job as a National Account Manager with Office Depot. Four months after my injury, I went back to work. The company and my customers were fully supportive of me from the beginning. There was no expectation that I would pick up where I left off. The first several weeks I worked a minimal schedule and gradually eased back into a normal routine. I am also blessed in that I am able to do much of my work from home.

I was also lucky to already have a beautiful bride in my life. Marsha and I have been together since 1989 and married since 1996. While I suffered the injury physically, the emotional and psychological distress affects her as much as it does me. She went through as much pain, anger, and frustration as I did about my injury, and it was important for her to share all of her emotions and not suppress anything for my sake. Open communication was, and still is, vital to the health of our relationship.

There have been many issues and situations that we've had to deal with. Vacations for us used to be planned around the types of physical activities we liked or wanted to try, whereas now they're more passive and usually involve sightseeing. Career decisions have required a different approach. While I enjoy my job immensely, I had considered leaving to pursue a career coaching high school track and cross country. I know that I can still take that on, but the health benefits I have now are excellent, and I don't want that to change. I also know the compensation would be considerably less, and because of many of the non-covered medical expenses, we don't want to bear the burden a reduction in salary would bring.

By our accounts, the only thing missing in our lives before my injury was a family beyond the two of us and our dogs, Bubba and June. We had talked about starting a family when my injury occurred. While traditional methods will not work for us now, there are still many options available. In-vitro fertilization is the method that we are exploring now. If that does not work we have considered adoption. The love that we have to give would not be diminished because of a blood line.

Among the curses of a SCI is the amount of time now required to accomplish many of life's daily activities. Little things like getting dressed or getting in and out of a car used to be easy but now require more time and effort. Of course the biggest inconvenience, and time consumer, is the bowel program. Beyond that, I have experimented and developed ways to save time in other areas.

To save time on laundry days, I will start a load of wash before I make breakfast. After I am done with breakfast, the clothes are ready for the dryer and I then start another load of wash. I then do my bowel routine so that when I am finished there are warm clothes waiting to be folded and put away.

While the above deals with life inside the house and the challenges faced, the outside world is equally daunting. Physical barriers are usually overcome with ramps, curb cuts, and good parking spots. Interaction with people, as SCI veterans can attest, is another game, even among friends and family.

My personal experience is that most people are unsure how to act around a wheelchair user; before my injury I was, too. As an able-bodied person, my uneasiness stemmed from not knowing the mindset of the person in the chair. Did they have feelings of anger and sadness, or were they just going about their day like me? I now try to make eye contact with people I encounter directly and offer the first greeting or acknowledgement.

Many of the people I deal with on a regular basis, impressed that I am usually in high spirits, praise me for my positive outlook. Do the words "heroic" and "inspirational" sound familiar? While those are well-meaning words, I usually interpret it as someone saying, "I'm glad it's you and not me."

For me, a hero is someone who makes a choice to help someone else without regard to his own well-being. Firefighters and rescue workers at the World Trade Center on September 11 are heroes, not me. What choice did I have to make? Live with my spinal cord injury or die. While I suppose it could have been an possibility via Dr. Jack Kevorkian, death was not an option for me. I suspect too that, given the choice, the people who perished in the attacks of September 11 would be willing to trade places with me.

While I think it's an overused phrase, we really are the ones in control of our happiness. Every day I find myself teetering between happiness and sadness, bitterness, anger, etc. There are so many reminders of a life that I no longer know or may never know: seeing people running or biking, fathers giving their kids a piggy-back ride, or doing any of the things that I can no longer do. When I'm in that situation, I have to remind myself that none of those things are what influences the love and support I get from my family and friends.

There are days when all I do is think about my old life to the point that I am totally consumed by bitterness. All that does though is waste the positive energy that I can direct toward other things or people. I am more conscious about that now and have fewer days of prolonged depression. Not that I have any experience, but I would assume it's like fighting an addiction to alcohol or drugs, and the best approach is to take one day at a time.

Not that I won't allow myself to think about the better days of the past. Many times when I am lying in bed, I will think about hiking or running with Marsha and the dogs. Because I am in bed and not in my chair, those images seem more real. There's also the hope that someday I may walk again and will have a chance to do those things I love so much.

I believe our attitude is the compass that guides our lives. I believe there is a God and that He guides us in our journey. I further believe that He doesn't know how our individual stories end and that our choices in life are not predetermined. I also have a deep-rooted fear that by taking anything in life for granted I may wind up with those things taken from me for good. Is that why I ended up like this in the first place? I don't think so.

I was, and still am, grateful for all the life I have. Why, then, did it happen? Who knows? I can recall many events in the past where through my negligence or someone else's, I escaped serious and possibly fatal injuries. Maybe the paralysis is mild compared to some other, and much worse, fate. I'm not sure. But, as I toe the line between happiness and sadness, for now, I choose happiness.

Mark Edwards lives in Fullerton, California, with his wife, Marsha, and their two dogs, Bubba and June. He is a national account manager with Office Depot and a volunteer with the American Cancer Society. While no longer hiking, mountain biking, or running, Mark enjoys handcycling, attempting to play the piano, and the occasional poker game.

No Barriers

Leslie Sward Greer
T12-L1
Age at SCI: 28
Date of SCI: August 12, 1989
Allen, Texas

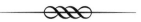

I became paraplegic at T12-L1 in August 1989, in an automobile accident where the lap belt held me firmly in place, but the shoulder harness was defective. The difference between the two snapped my back.

I was twenty-eight, married, and had a two-year-old son sleeping in his car seat in the back of the car. My husband, David, was driving; I was the front passenger. We were on our way to Destin, Florida, for a much needed family vacation. In Mississippi, on a stretch of the interstate with no shoulder to the road and the trees lining the highway, a tie rod apparently broke under our car. While my husband was standing on the brakes and yanking the steering wheel to the left, we headed to the right and hit a tree.

Thankfully, our son flew out of his car seat and onto my lap in the front seat without a scratch. My husband lost a few teeth and broke his ankle kicking out the door to get out of the car. I had a huge knot on my forehead from shattering the front windshield and excruciating back pain.

After surgery and a two-week stint in Mississippi, I was flown back to Dallas to begin rehabilitation. I had a lovely hard plastic body cast on that was extremely hot and itchy. As I was wheeled through the rehabilitation hospital, it rode up so that it looked as if my chest and neck were glued together. The best part about the cast was that I had the firmest boobs in town for the three months I wore it! At night, when I was in bed and promised not to move, the nurses would undo the Velcro straps and let me open the shell I was encased in so I could scratch to my heart's content. That was the best part of my day.

Rehabilitation was a long, hard road designed to make me as independent as possible. When they attempted to teach me to vacuum and cook, I refused, saying, "I didn't do those things before my accident. What makes you think I want to do them now?" They laughed and taught me anyway.

Since my husband travels for his job about three weeks each month, he never knew that I had learned how to do household chores. About three years later, I decided that our living room needed cleaning and was vacuuming away, when I heard the back door open unexpectedly. I wheeled around and there he was — with his arms crossed, looking at me — dumbfounded. I have been paying penance ever since. He actually bought me a self-propelled vacuum one Christmas. How thoughtful!

Living with a disability is not what I had imagined. A few days after back surgery, my caseworker at the hospital asked me to critique a book on spinal cord injury that the hospital had compiled. Bored to tears just lying there and unable to move because I did not have a functioning body, I agreed to look over the book and make suggestions. Although the book was fairly elementary in scope, it sure opened my eyes as to what lay ahead. The part about internal organs being paralyzed from your point of injury, sometimes upwards and definitely downwards, certainly caught my attention.

That meant my bladder, my bowels, my female parts, and my private parts. The idea that my private parts would no longer have feeling had my head spinning. They tried to tell me that good sex was a cerebral function — that feeling came from my brain. However, that was not the area of my anatomy that had previously had that feeling. It wasn't my brain that had glowed after good sex. How could they say that?

I had no idea that my total body would be affected. I thought it was just my limbs and my muscles, not my internal organs. I imagined I was going to look like some poster child for paraplegics, with various apparatus stuck on my body, saying, "Oh, please excuse my urine sack hanging off the end of my wheelchair. This doesn't turn you off does it?" If we can send a man to the moon and drop a bomb with pinpoint accuracy, shouldn't there be some creative devices that allow bodily functions to happen without the use of latex gloves, tubes, catheters, or plastic bags?

While in rehab I met Lydia. She had jumped off some cliffs into a lake and broken her back also at T12-L1. We became roommates and found that we had many similar attitudes. After a grueling day of physical or occupational therapy, we would talk into the night discussing how we experienced the doctors and other professionals as very negative. We had both been positive people before our accidents and had families that were verbally pushing us to get better, grow from the experience, and move on. We did not want to let ourselves believe that we were not going to get better.

After hearing from doctors, nurses, and behavioral medicine specialists — who were supposed to be helping us — that we were going to have to accept the fact that we would never walk again, my husband would probably divorce me, Lydia's boyfriend would ditch her, we would never have children, we would have difficulty finding a job, and our friends would stop coming around, we got really mad. We decided to take our healing into our own hands. That's when life started to go better for us. We were not willing to give up our lives and sit around feeling sorry for ourselves.

Taking charge was the smartest thing we ever did. No more pills to keep us sedated or quiet so that we might not have the nerve to question what was being done to us. We got strong mentally, and that, in turn, helped us physically. We soared from there. We didn't need colostomies or drugs to help us cope. To our great delight, we found out that good sex really is a cerebral function. There are many ways to enjoy sex, and we found out just how creative we could be. We were shown movies on various positions and techniques we could try, which can be embarrassing when you are sitting in a room with thirty people you don't know. Most people went home and practiced with their significant other in their own bed. However, I do know of a woman who went out and bought five different kinds of vibrating devices to see which one might work. No telling what the store clerk thought when she was purchasing all these items at once. That sort of sexual experimentation is trial and error and sometimes downright hilarious.

Two weeks after leaving the hospital, I threw myself into society again and forced myself to learn how to do things differently. I went back to work where, fortunately, my job as a credit manager and human resource manager for a telecommunications company was completely accessible. I just got a better parking space.

I didn't use a power chair because I needed the exercise. I wheeled around everywhere with my two-year-old son on my lap. When I went shopping, I held him while pushing a cart full of groceries. If I really got rolling down an aisle and realized that I could not stop, we would just crash into a store display and laugh. If I was in bed or sitting on the sofa, Christian took great pleasure in stealing my wheelchair and taking it for a spin around the house or coasting down the driveway. He always forgot to bring it back. I was always calling my neighbor and asking her to go on a search and rescue mission. I wouldn't trade those memories for anything.

A few years after my accident, I gave birth to another son. I now have two fine boys — one who knew me slightly before the accident and one who has not known me any other way.

In May 1997, Lydia graduated from law school. As we were discussing the barriers we encountered while we were trying to be independent, we focused on restaurants and businesses that had poor parking, difficult paths of travel, steep ramps, narrow doorways, inaccessible restrooms, etc. It was getting increasingly frustrating that, although the ADA had been signed several years earlier, we did not have independent access to many places of business. If we were fortunate enough to get a parking space, there was no ramp. If we got in the doors, we could not use a bathroom because there was no getting through a stall door.

We knew we wanted to do something that would benefit the community to give back for the nice things that were done for us by strangers — who came in to just say hello, bring our family food, give us a friendly smile. We formed No Barriers, Inc., a not-for-profit corporation, to assist businesses in removing architectural barriers and making their facilities accessible. No Barriers has been quite successful, and we continue to help the disability community gain access to places that were previously "off limits."

My identity as a person has changed somewhat. I am more humbled by life's experiences. I try to smile more and frown less. I take time to notice things that I just didn't pay attention to or have the time for. I had been concentrating on being upwardly mobile in a career. Now, I am just concerned with being mobile in a manual chair! Before my accident, I had never been on a job interview where I wasn't offered something. Afterward, I withstood rejections and, for the first time, felt what it was like to be perceived as "different." I don't mind when children stare. After all, they are just trying to learn. I don't want them to be afraid of a wheelchair or me; I always try to answer questions and joke around to make them feel comfortable.

When my children bring friends over, one of their favorite activities is to play in my elevator. It has a telephone, and they think it is their own personal telephone booth. Once, the electricity in our house went out and I got stuck between floors. My youngest son, Richard, was about four at the time and was downstairs diligently watching cartoons. I yelled for him to please go and push the emergency release so that I could get back to the bottom floor. His response was "I can't!" "Why not?" "I'm watching Scooby Doo, Mommy!" I called a neighbor.

I've been rerouted on my path through life, but my heart is still the same. I still love children and animals, and since my children sometimes act like animals, this works out well. I still have soft spots for my mom and dad and my husband and kids. I thank them, in my thoughts, every night for pushing me to not be a quitter and for daring me to learn something new. As often as possible, I thank them verbally. I still have the people who were truly my friends before the accident, and I have been fortunate enough to make some new friends. My disability has brought me into contact with people that I may never have had the opportunity to meet. I end my day feeling good, knowing that I tried to help others gain access. I am being included and not excluded, and I assist others in doing the same.

I still have the same wonderful husband and two wonderful sons. I still vacuum and clean, darn it. I drive my car with hand controls and take great pride into swinging into a disabled parking space near the front door of the mall at Christmas when everyone else has to take the shuttle in. I am quite adept at carrying packages on my lap with their handles grasped firmly between my teeth. If I ever need dentures, this could pose a problem, but for now I'm safe. I push a grocery cart because I am not allowed to use the store's electric scooter model since I once knocked over a display using it. If my children talk back, I pop a wheelie and land the front wheels on their toes. They have become perfect children!

I begin each day appreciating life. I try to laugh at life's glitches because that is what I choose to do. I've always used that approach because my parents taught me that life is worth appreciating. I am having fun and enjoying life, not just existing. If they finally find a cure for spinal cord injury, I'm not sure what I will do. If I get back my ability to ambulate, what will happen to my parking space?

Leslie Sward Greer lives in Allen, Texas. She has been married nineteen years and has two sons. She works as the accounting manager for the City of Allen Police Department. During the evening hours and weekends, she spends time with her family and working as the president of No Barriers, Inc.

Finding the Cure on the Inside

Michael Hurlock
C4-5
Age at SCI: 18
Date of SCI: July 17, 1990
Chaplin, Connecticut

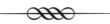

O n July 17, 1990, I was working at the summer recreation camp for the town of Mansfield, Connecticut. I was eighteen, about a month removed from my high school graduation, destined for college. While helping supervise the seventh and eighth grade group at the town's public swimming pond, I decided to take off my shoes and socks and join the kids in the water.

I ran along the beach, taking two or three steps into the water, and then dove in, as I'd done a hundred times before. My head must have been tilted a little too far forward, causing it to hit bottom, instantly paralyzing me at C4-5. Ironically, there was an emergency water safety class on the other side of the pond that was practicing the very rescue techniques they were suddenly asked to put to real use.

As I lay face down in the water, totally numb, a serene calmness came over me. It was not my life that flashed before my eyes — but my future. My college career at Rutgers University — gone. My ability to play basketball and other sports — gone. My positive body image — gone. The confidence to ask an attractive woman out — gone. Walking down the aisle with a future bride — gone. My life as I knew it — all seemingly gone.

The shock really hit me in intensive care when a nurse was lifting something in the air, and then I realized it was my arm! I could not believe it — no sensation at all. I wanted an alien ship to beam me up and take me back in time to just before the accident.

All I knew about spinal cord injuries was what I had seen on television and in movies — people paralyzed "from the waist down." So after a couple of days, I changed my thinking to where I could accept not being able to use my legs. It's like I was bargaining with God — you can have my legs, but just let me be able to use my arms. Just two weeks earlier I had bought my first CD player, and I desperately wanted to be able to change the discs myself.

After a couple of weeks, with no further improvement in my arms, and an over-abundance of free time spent hoping, obsessing, and praying in my rotating hospital bed, I realized there would be no bargaining. I'd lost almost all of my hope, became depressed, and actually imagined what it would be like to end my life. Then I was laughing at the irony of not being physically able to do it on my own.

Five weeks later I was rehabbing at Craig Hospital near Denver, learning ways to manage my bladder and bowels, increase my breathing capacity after I got off the respirator, protect my skin from breakdown, and to drive a wheelchair with a sip and puff control. I desperately wanted to gain enough arm strength to drive a joystick-controlled chair because it looked more "normal." It took a couple of weeks — not to mention a couple of crashes — to accept that sip and puff was how I would be getting around.

My friend John lived in Denver and spent time watching Monday night football with me, while my dad, mom, brother, and sister visited at various times from Connecticut for a couple of days at a time. My mom stayed for the entire last month of my rehab to learn about my personal care so that we could all be ready for the transition out into the "real world."

I was leaving a fully accessible place where I had help from numerous staff and was accepted by everyone there. I returned to a world that is generally inaccessible, and where I imagined being discriminated against and stared at like some sort of freak. I was scared out of my mind again.

All of my friends had gone off to college. My fraternal twin brother was in New Hampshire enjoying the adventures of a college freshman, while I was still getting used to a body that no longer worked on its own. It was hard to see my twin having the experiences I would never get to share — a constant reminder of what my life might have been like.

The doctors in both Hartford and Denver told me that the spinal cord cure was probably just five or ten years away. I thought that if I could just get through a couple of years, then a cure would come along and I could be my old self again. I believe this made my transition much more difficult, because acceptance was not possible. I became obsessed with trying to maintain my body in ways that would preserve it for the soon-to-arrive cure. Every half-hour I would ask someone to reposition me if my body did not look quite right.

That March on spring break in Miami, my brother learned of a potential "breakthrough" with rats and mice at The Miami Project To Cure Paralysis. They projected perhaps seven or eight years before it would be available. My future orientation on life and a cure began to slowly crash. I saw that these doctors had no idea when any sort of cure would happen. It was just something to say.

On my first Christmas home from rehab I received two gifts — a computer game, and the book "Misery" by my favorite author, Stephen King — that made me furious, although I didn't show it. How was I supposed to use these gifts? I had been listening to books on tape because I couldn't turn the pages, let alone use the keyboard to play the computer game.

Gradually, these two gifts began to have a positive effect. I was sick of knowing the soap opera story lines, and took no pride in how adept I'd become at "The Price Is Right." So my parents and I began to improvise. We used pillows and a tray to put the keyboard at a height that allowed me to type using a mouthstick. The same thing worked with books! Soon I had a desk I could roll up to for computing and reading as I desired. I felt more in control — which helped my self-esteem and changed my negative world-view. My confidence soared, and by that summer I felt ready for the University of Connecticut.

The freedom of my power chair, my new van, and starting college slowly made it clear to me that having a life now, as I was, had no effect whatsoever on my potential to be "cured." Although I still do things like use a standing frame and a functional electrical stimulation bike, I am more realistic about the possibility for cure. If one comes, that's great. In the meantime, I'm going to live my life.

No longer able to compete at a physical level, my drive changed to doing my best at an academic level. I completely threw myself into my studies and excelled, even as I felt so different from everyone else in my classes. During discussions, I did not contribute much because I could not raise my hand. I was not the type to just speak up and interrupt, although occasionally I did. It was also embarrassing to make an announcement during the first class of the semester asking if someone could take notes for me. When the class was over, I would wait as people walked by to see who would volunteer their services. On one occasion, no one volunteered and I had to make the same announcement before the next class. I felt like a charity case.

Sprinkle in a little personal psychotherapy for myself while adjusting to my new identity, an introductory psychology course, and bingo — my career path came to life. I had found a way to help others in the same ways that so many have helped me. I graduated in the spring of 1995 with a bachelor's degree in psychology, a master's degree in counseling psychology in 1998, and then a master's degree in marriage and family therapy in 2000. I'm now in the doctoral program for marriage and family therapy at the University of Connecticut, one of the top programs in the country.

Being in charge of my own personal care is difficult. It's like running a business. I am in charge of payroll, hiring and interviewing new attendants, and firing them when they don't meet my standards for promptness and responsibility. Just when everything seems to be in perfect harmony, it's almost guaranteed that something in the system will fail. This constant reminder of my dependence on people and on machines humbles me. I used to worry so much about the things that could happen — and set me back for days, or even weeks — that I would hesitate to take on more responsibility in school, work — and even love. I was afraid of letting everyone down if I couldn't follow through.

But if I were not in charge of my own personal care, then my control over my life would diminish down to nothing, and that's called a "nursing home." Now I have about eight attendants working for me — most of them very wonderful people. They have helped me increase my control over my environment. I have a sense of being in charge. I could not possibly list the many ways they help me. As wonderful as they are, I cherish the time I can be left alone without them there to remind me of my dependence.

Sometimes I drive myself too hard and expect too much of myself. During one of my internships, I was the only one that didn't miss a day of work either semester, yet I still worried that my spinal cord injury "baggage" would screw things up. People have things happen to them all the time — whether they have a spinal cord injury or not. I just know that I work ten times as hard as the next person, trying to prove myself, because society expects me to fail. My drive comes from wanting to prove society wrong — a drive that is sometimes too strong for my own good. I'm still learning to give myself a break.

I'm disturbed by the subtle ways people treat me differently. People who are uncomfortable when they first meet me either treat me like I am mentally retarded or they avoid interacting with me at all — costing them the chance to get to know me. I was initially very reserved when meeting new people, feeling anxious about the assumptions I thought they might be making about me. Most of the time, I would wait for people to approach me first.

I'm more comfortable with myself now. When I meet people for the first time I think, "Fuck it, I'm going to be myself and not let their anxiety affect me." I've learned to be more myself while educating others. Whenever I get the chance to tell my story, I do so gladly. I try to be open and honest so people can know me for the person I am.

I'll never forget the date of July 17th. My spinal cord injury was a tragic event, but it was also a rebirth. My injury has led me to mature quick-

ly and to look at life very differently. I'm proud of the many positive qualities it's given me. If I actually had the choice to go back and change things,
it would be difficult — more and more so with each positive experience.

With my injury — and perhaps because of it — my life has meaning
and purpose. If I can use my experiences to help others find meaning and
purpose in their lives, then any bitterness that I might have left about my situation becomes a little sweeter, and my acceptance a little easier. I don't know
if I would have that if I not been injured. I thought I switched from one identity to another after my injury — and in some ways I have — but in the most
important ways I'm the same person.

*Mike Hurlock lives in Chaplin, Connecticut. He is a doctoral student at
the University of Connecticut in the School of Family Studies. He works part time
at both the University's Family Center and at the Alcohol and Other Drug Education Center as a therapist/counselor. He is a popular speaker on campus regarding sexuality and disability, and is a huge college basketball and pro football fan.*

Back on the Dance Floor of Life

Bobbie Humphreys
C5-6
Age at SCI: 17
Date of SCI: April 17, 1973
Parsippany, New Jersey

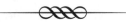

*I*n northern New Jersey where I grew up, we were twelve brothers, sisters, and cousins — competitive as well as supportive of each other. We camped, skied, and were involved in school sports and/or played musical instruments. I started dating in seventh grade and had many different boyfriends. In April 1973, I was seventeen, a junior in high school, and captain of the field hockey team when I brought an old boyfriend to a local dirt-bike track where he could ride his 250 Kawasaki. My two older brothers had motorcycles, so they were not foreign to me. After riding around doing some jumps, my boyfriend talked me into giving it a try. "I'll do this just once," I thought. Wearing sneakers, jeans, and a helmet, I revved the engine, felt very excited, and tried to remember everything he had said to do in order to jump the bike correctly. But, I forgot to lift the handlebars up!

Everything began moving in slow motion. Somehow, I knew that I would break my neck. I just wasn't sure if I would die instantly or be paralyzed for life. I heard my neck break, and my body fell to the ground like a rag doll.

I took control of my situation immediately, calmed everyone, and instructed the paramedic to "be careful how you remove my helmet, or you'll kill me." Then I introduced myself to break the tension.

My first concern was "nobody will want to take me to the senior prom." After six weeks in Krutchfield tongs traction, I had surgery to fuse my spine together for stabilization. Then, I waited for a bed at Kessler Institute for Rehabilitation, ten miles from my home. When my parents wanted to send me to an "institute," I thought they were sending me away for good. I had screwed up big time; this was my punishment.

At Kessler, I was overwhelmed by how many young people were in wheelchairs. I had never seen a young person in a wheelchair. I hated it because I saw myself in them, and I didn't like what I saw — young people, broken and crippled. After I got to know the individuals in the wheelchairs, I realized that they were just as scared and confused as I was about sex, marriage, work, and the future. They, too, had parents, brothers, sisters, and friends who were affected by their injuries.

I felt lucky with my C5-6 level of injury compared to people like Butchy who couldn't move his arms, feed himself, wipe a tear, or give a hug. I was nick-named "Super Quad" because I had the use of the triceps muscle in my right arm. My peers were my sounding board, and self-pity was not allowed. It was useless to complain about having calluses on my hands from pushing on the tires of the wheelchair to those who couldn't move their arms.

The support of my family was a huge positive factor. But family and friends didn't visit as often as I'd hoped. I needed them to be there to see my latest accomplishment — writing my name in script instead of block letters. Later, I learned that they were afraid of saying the wrong thing, like, "Do you want to go outside for a walk?" They thought I would burst into tears if they said "walk" or "run."

Discharged after five months, I didn't get the welcome home party I had anticipated. I was flooded with mixed emotions. With the unconditional support of my hospital peers, I had been adapting somewhat okay. But, at home, my family couldn't and didn't understand what I was adjusting to. I got angry with them for not being able to read my mind, and started abusing them by cursing them out. Unknowingly, I was angry with them for being able to do everyday tasks that now took me hours. They just took them for granted. How dare they!

At Kessler, I had gotten used to everything being flat, sterile, white, and noisy. Now, I was mystified by the different smells and colors and how deafeningly quiet the house was. No longer were there changing shifts of nurses and aides to help me with my many daily needs — just my scared, newly trained mother and two younger sisters. Patti helped me with everything and anything I asked without question. But, my younger sister, Dee Dee, always said, "Try it yourself first. If you can't do it, I'll help." At the time, I thought she was being mean and lazy. In the long run, she helped me more by making me try — even when it took me an hour of tears to make a peanut butter and jelly sandwich.

My parents had separated while I was in the hospital. Since my dad and I had disagreed frequently, mostly about my choices of boyfriends, I thought I would love getting my way, and that the house would be quieter. I missed my dad's presence far more that I had anticipated. It made me sad. Was it my fault that my parents had separated? I had sensed that there had been tension between my parents. My accident was not the underlying cause of their separation.

With my sisters in school and mom at work, I finished high school at home via an intercom system. Spending a lot of time alone, I became very depressed. What would I do for a living? How could I contribute to society? I felt totally useless, especially without the use of my hands. How could I possibly drive a car? If I couldn't drive, how would I get places? I no longer wanted to talk, eat, or drink — just cry and sleep. The accident only took one second but it changed my life forever. Why me? Was I being punished? These thoughts consumed me constantly. I could not see any purpose to my life — just despair. I couldn't imagine marriage, children, a house, working, or even having fun.

My sisters, cousins, and friends felt my doom, and intervened. They took turns getting me up out of bed, out of the house, and back out on the dance floor. For every negative thought I had about my physical or mental limitations, they had their usual "got to be a way" attitude. They snapped me out of my private pity party. My family never tolerated whining. To them, my disability challenge was no different. If I would get down or cry, my sisters or cousins would say, "Let's go out dancing. You will have fun." They did not see that I had a disability. I was just the same old Bobbie they still loved very much. And, I went to my senior prom!

After my discharge, I believed that if I only had able-bodied friends, I would be less disabled. If I looked into a mirror or at another person using a wheelchair, I would have to face my "problem." I decided to ignore my disability by not acknowledging it. I even refused to use any adaptive device that would make life easier because it would make me look and feel handicapped.

At two years post, I heard "Shower the People," a song by James Taylor, "Shower the people you love with love. Show them the way that you feel. Things will work out fine, if you want they will." I started projecting a positive attitude everywhere. If I went out, I would make eye contact, smile, and say a cheerful hello to anybody, especially strangers — and they always smiled back. As my new attitude and outlook changed, so did the way people saw and treated me. My positive attitude was bouncing back at me! I realized how an attitude, good or bad, can be powerful and contagious.

I began doing more around the house, getting out, and meeting people. As I became happier, I found I liked being around myself, too. I got hooked on all the fun and life that had continued while I was away. My pre-injury serial monogamous dating picked back up. I was alive, healthy, and lucky.

I also discovered a new breed of men who "enjoyed" dating women who were physically dependent on them. Beware — there are some men and women in this world who "get off" on having total and complete control over another person's body. I learned that whenever I sensed an uneasy feeling about a person, I needed to listen to my inner voice.

I attended Ramapo College, where I lived on campus and discovered my love for music and theatre. Living on my own, I was forced to supervise my own home health care. I learned what I could and couldn't do for myself. I found that asking for help was okay — people like to help. I began to have greater respect for myself and others, and became less selfish. My SCI affected everyone around me, and a whole new appreciation emerged for my family and friends. I blossomed and accepted my challenge instead of fighting it. I even did laundry for able-bodied students for extra money.

During the summer of 1980, seven years post, I got a van equipped for me to drive. My sister Patti and I drove ten thousand miles across the United States, camping the whole way, doing cath changes and bowel programs in a tent. I never thought, "How are we going to do this?" I thought, "How can we not do it?" Traveling across the country had always been a dream — why should my injury change that? In Montana, we met up with some friends and decided to go to the top of Hidden Lake, ninety-five hundred feet up. The four of them took turns pushing me to the top. Sitting on top of the mountain in Glacier National Park, I felt anything was possible. It brought to mind the words on a little figurine given to me while I was still in traction, "Always take on more than you can possibly handle, or you'll never be able to do all that you can do."

Nine years post, I met Pete, a most extraordinary, compassionate man. Pete fell in love at first sight with Bobbie, the woman, looking past my wheelchair. We met in a biker bar. It took Pete another ten days to track me down to ask me out. Our first date was at a dance club. When Pete asked me if I wanted to dance and what he should do to dance with me, I lowered my armrest to my lap level and told him to put most of his weight on the armrest and start dancing. We held each other and rocked to the music. After a slow dance and talking until 2 a.m., we've been together ever since. Personality-wise, we are total opposites — Pete is the quiet, stay-at-home type — yet we provide each other with a great balance. Pete is also a trained home health care aide who provides a hundred percent of my care with gentle ease.

In 1976, remembering my stay at Kessler when my peers and I wished there had been seasoned people with spinal cord injuries to answer our many questions, I felt a peer counseling program would be invaluable. When I approached the administration, they did not see the necessity of it. Finally, in 1991, after lobbying the administration for over fifteen years, I was successful, and the peer counseling program at Kessler began. Although the program was for people with recent injuries, I became one of its beneficiaries. I hadn't thought I'd have to talk about myself or my own personal feelings — just tell people how I did things. Answering questions forced me to deal with my own issues. I hadn't realized that I was still in denial about being disabled until they asked me how I dealt with my denial. Facing those questions was very tough. The program helped me acknowledge issues I had pushed to the back of my mind, like how hearing my family talk about skiing and camping trips and the fun they had that I could no longer experience really did bother me.

As I interacted in peer counseling sessions, I learned about the stages of grief people go through when they lose the ability to walk — denial, isolation, anger, bargaining, depression, and acceptance — and saw how my experience fit these stages.

I became aware of my own denial through the peer program. I remembered the isolation I experienced when I was on my own, alone in the house. After I was home for about a year, I had expressed my anger by verbally abusing the people closest to me. Fortunately, I realized that being angry pushed people away, and I changed back to the more considerate person I had been. I was bargaining when I was experimenting with alcohol and drugs and rationalized by telling myself I would continue until my body was cured. To this day, I still deal with depression. In the beginning, it was about walking, then sexual frustration. Now, it's watching my sisters and cousins living "normal" lives with their spouses and children, houses and jobs.

When I was first injured, I believed I would never amount to anything or contribute to society in a productive way. After thirty years, I am much more patient with myself and others. I totally gave up hoping for a cure years ago. Living is more important than the act of walking. As long as I am productive through working part-time or volunteering, and learning needlepoint, calligraphy, quilting, and singing in a symphonic choir, I feel content. Currently I'm working on an autobiography and still do peer counseling. I'm very grateful and fortunate for the support of family and friends, Pete, our apartment, and a van I can drive. I am living a full life.

Bobbie Humphreys lives in Parsippany, New Jersey. She is a peer counselor at Kessler Institute for Rehabilitation and has volunteered at several nonprofit organizations. Currently, she is writing her autobiography, doing a woodwork art project, and singing in a symphonic concert choir.

Hunting More Than Ever

Breck Lonier
T5
Age at SCI: 36
Date of SCI: October 4, 1999
Lansing, Michigan

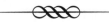

I grew up in the country and love the outdoors — hunting, fishing, landscaping, and lifting weights during the winter months. On my mother's birthday, October 4, 1999, while I was hunting deer with a bow, I fell 14 feet from a tree injuring my spinal cord at the T5 level.

I don't remember the fall. All I can remember is waking up able to move only my arms and head, and seeing my family standing around me. I knew in that moment that my life was going to take a drastic change for the worse.

After my surgery, I spent two months in Mary Free Bed in Grand Rapids, Michigan, for rehabilitation. The nurses and therapists were outstanding. They enabled me to get on with the physical aspects of my life, and allowed me to feel the emotions that I needed to feel — up or down. If I'm having a bad day, the last thing I want is for someone to tell me, "Oh, it's not that bad."

Leaving rehab was scary after being used to someone always being there to take care of me. Since I had a lot of visitors, I was alone very little to sit and think about how my life was going to change. Once I got home, the changes became very overwhelming. I had to move in with my mother for three weeks until the modifications to my house were completed. I began to question whether or not I wanted to live this way.

We tore down the old garage and built a new one with a ramp into the house, converted one bedroom into a large bathroom, widened all the doorways, and modified the sink in the kitchen. It was not much different than being in the hospital. Mom waited on me hand and foot, which all moms would do.

During that time, my ex-wife brought my son, Garrett, to visit me, as she did while I was in rehab. Renee has always encouraged me to be a part of his life, talking about how much he needed me. He was only four and a half, and did not understand that I could not get out of my chair. He kept asking me to get on the floor and play with him and do things that I could not do. It was all I could do not to cry.

After he left, I felt like a failure as a father and thought he would be better off without me as a burden in his life. For several days, I kept thinking about this and how it would be better to die. I had a huge supply of pain killers and figured that if I took a lot of them, they would kill me and it would be over. I waited until my mom went back to work — her first day to leave me alone — and then I took them. Fortunately for me, they just made me really sick.

I obviously needed to talk to someone about all my feelings, so Mom found a psychologist who specialized in rehabilitation patients. I had a lot in common with him — he liked hunting and fishing, too. It helped talking to him, but what really made a difference was just time and adjusting to my new life.

On New Years Eve, 1999, I moved back into my house — alone. In the beginning, my mother had a hard time with me living on my own. Once she saw that I could do it, she began to relax. Since I knew I was going to be stuck for at least two months because I was not able to drive yet, I had a satellite dish installed and signed up for all the movie channels. But just sitting around in front of the television can be depressing, so I had to find a hobby. I used to enjoy drawing and had done a few wood-burning pictures when I was about nineteen years old, so I started working on wood burnings while I watched movies. It helped keep my mind off how miserable I thought my life was.

I had quit taking my pain pills because I didn't want to get addicted to them. After I stopped taking them I started sweating and had the chills all the time. I was also having trouble with urinary tract infections and my bowel movements. One day I was so depressed that I wanted to try to commit suicide again, but I told myself to wait until tomorrow to see how I would feel. And no matter how bad things were, I knew I still had a responsibility to my son.

The next day I woke up and felt good, anxious to get back to the wood-burning picture I was working on. From that day on every time I was depressed or felt like I was ready to give up I would just say to myself, "Wait until tomorrow." Crying also helped. Sometimes, I would cry until I could not cry anymore — just got it out of my system — and would feel a lot better. Deep down inside I guess I realized that it would get better and I needed to take it one day at a time. I had a choice of sitting around being depressed or moving on. I chose to move on.

I went to a family doctor to see if he could find out why I was always sweating and cold. He gave me some non-addictive pills to try. I took two of them and about an hour later I wasn't sweating anymore. I also learned that I was not drinking enough water. My urinary tract infections went away after I made a habit of drinking a half gallon of water every morning on an empty stomach. It only takes me about 20 minutes to drink all of it. I drink another quart of water at around four in the afternoon. I found that if I drank too much water close to bedtime there was a good chance of getting wet in my sleep!

It took about six months to figure out how to manage my bowel movements. I'm not able to tell when I'm going to have one, and have had to make a mad rush to my toilet chair, literally cut off my underwear, and wait for the process to be over. Sometimes, I would wake up in the morning and find one helluva mess to clean up.

Until I came across a book about spinal cord injuries that explained how to use my finger and slowly make a circular motion to relax the muscles and allow for easier bowel movements. I started doing this every other day at about the same time, and it seems to work well. As time went by, I was able to understand my body and what it was trying to tell me.

This helped a lot with my depression and being able to go places with friends. Once or twice a week, I would get a ride to the shop of a friend of mine who is a taxidermist to help him out. It felt good to get out of my house for a while. The only thing that seemed to depress me a little were sunny days. All I could think about was what I would be doing if I weren't in this damned chair.

I vowed to myself that I would not go back to work until I could drive myself there. First, I had to take driving lessons so I could get a license to drive with hand controls. Then, I had to wait for the state to provide funding for the conversions to my truck. Finally, my truck was converted and I returned to my job as a supervisor in a small steel fabrication plant on May 1, 2000, after being gone for seven months. My supervisors had been very much a part of my rehabilitation. They visited me often, encouraged me to come back to work, and accepted me without any doubt that I would be able to do my job. The first day back was great! Everyone was happy to see me. My disability insurance company wanted me to slowly work my way up to an eight-hour day, but I didn't want to leave at the end of the day. I worked for eight hours on the first day and never looked back.

Once I returned to work my back felt better. When I was sitting home doing wood burnings, my back would tighten up and the spasms in my legs would increase. At work the spasms went away. My back is always in some pain, but is not nearly as bad when I do a lot of moving around. I usually wait until the weekend to clean the floors and do the laundry.

Once my truck was converted, I started spending more time with Garrett, now six years old. I found that we could do a lot of things together — fishing, the movies, playing board games. That season I took him hunting with me for his first time. We were watching some does, fawns, and some turkeys when a small buck came out into the clover field. I told my son that we couldn't shoot him because he was too small. He looked at me and asked, "You can't shoot him because you don't have a small buck license?"

"Yes," I said, not knowing whether to laugh or cry. "I only have a big buck license!" About a half-hour later we shot a good-sized buck with my crossbow. That day made me realize that my life was worth living and my son was one of the best reasons I had to go on living. It made a huge difference in my outlook when I realized that I could be a great dad even without being able to walk or run with him.

Hunting in my new lifestyle has been very successful. I'd made a special set of arms for the bow and my gun that allowed me to shoot very effectively from my chair. The only problem I had was staying warm and having to rely on someone to drop me off and pick me up at my tent blind — a structure hunters use to wait for deer without being visible. The following year I designed a blind with a ramp that was insulated and big enough for two people. My cousins and friends helped me build it. I ran cables through pulleys to the Plexiglas windows so that I could open any of them from one spot. I converted a golf cart, adding hand controls, a harness seat belt, and a small platform on the side for my wheelchair. The cart doesn't scare the deer at all. I've hunted more the last two years than ever.

I still live alone with my dogs, a beagle and a black lab. I cook my own meals, and converted my riding lawn mower so I can mow the lawn. Sometimes when I go to a store and other places, people try and help me do things. I always let them. Not that I need help, but I think it makes them feel good.

I realize now that instead of feeling sorry for myself and thinking that I would never be able to do the things that I enjoyed, I should have been focusing on trying to do them in a different way. I think a lot of people spend too much time wanting more, instead of just appreciating what they already have. They don't realize that at any time their lives could take a drastic change and all the money and toys in the world can't change it back.

So I've decided to live my new lifestyle. I truly feel that my life is good, I don't feel I am compromising anything. I make the most of what I have and can do. I am at peace with that. To dwell on the past gets me nowhere.

Breck Lonier lives in Lansing, Michigan. He is a manager at a steel manufacturing company.

A Search for Self–Worth

Kris Ann Piazza
C5
Age at SCI: 12
Date of SCI: June 24, 1980
Buffalo, New York

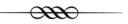

I was only twelve years old when my blossoming pre-teen independence was shattered by a rough shove from a schoolmate that sent
me plunging head first to the bottom of the pool. The impact broke
my fifth cervical vertebrae and caused irreparable damage to my spinal cord.

My life shuddered with shock, grinding to a halt while my family
rushed to my side to provide an emergency emotional backup system. The
scope of what was happening to my body was beyond my twelve-year-old
comprehension. I was terrified by an uncertain future and repulsed by my
inability to control such basics as bowel and bladder functions. One moment
I was pounding softballs into left field with my athletic body, and in the next
I found myself connected to a ventilator that was filling me with the breath
I could no longer bring to my own lungs.

Three days later I was off the ventilator, but who I had become — and
the loss of the person I thought I would never be — sickened me. Everyone
wanted me to fight, but I couldn't understand what I was supposed to be

fighting for. I had been athletic and independent, and none of that seemed possible any more. I wanted no part of the life I was enduring and selfishly tried to drag my family into the misery that was overwhelming me.

But they refused to go along, challenging me to reach for more than I was willing to believe was possible. I had chosen to hide in a dark hospital room, absorbed in my self-pity, refusing rehabilitation, until my sister shocked me with a good swift kick — emotionally — in the behind.

"I'm sick of watching you give up," she said, threatening to leave me to my misery if I didn't shape up.

I threw her out, saying, "I don't need you, and I'll be glad if you never come back!" It was the first serious fight we ever had. I was devastated, up all night thinking about our argument. But I knew in my heart she would come back, where she found me in my wheelchair, waiting. After tears of apology, relief, and joy, I made a serious commitment to rehab from that point on.

In 1980, there were no visible role models to reassure me that I could still have a meaningful life. There was no Internet abounding with stories of people succeeding with SCI. Christopher Reeve was still playing an indestructible Superman, and the Americans with Disabilities Act was a decade away. I was on my own, feeling mentally and physically immobilized.

I felt stuck in a box people placed me in, categorized and labeled disabled. I felt like nothing in society's eyes, which was a terrible blow for a twelve-year-old who already believed she was something. My high school years found me cowering in the shadows of perfect adolescent bodies that cast a dark cloud over my self-esteem. Many times, I fought back lonely tears while eavesdropping on conversations about the latest dance and who was going with whom. I wanted to be pursued by hormone-ridden boys and giggle about cute guys with my girlfriends, too.

I was becoming a young woman with a developing young woman's concerns, but asking questions about sex was taboo in my single-parent, Catholic home. No one was comfortable talking to me about sexuality except my former hospital roommate, and she thought the whole thing was a waste of time after paralysis. It all gave me the impression that paralyzed people were asexual and undesirable. I felt ugly and ashamed of my body, unable to explore my adolescence in a more positive light. It was as if my questions about becoming a woman embarrassed people — including the medical professionals and my family and friends. And that embarrassed me. I had a passionate nature that was demanding answers, but I had no one to turn to.

Control was another issue for me after the injury. I longed to feel in command of my life and inadvertently found a perverse kind of satisfaction in starvation as I turned fifteen. Choosing whether or not I fed my body when it was hungry was a powerful high. I went through years of unhealthy eating patterns trying to prove that I was the one in charge when anorexia was insidiously turning the tables on me. It took a serious toll on my mind and body. By the time I was nineteen, the eating disorder was full-blown. I developed common anorexic characteristics like perfectionism, body image distortion, malnutrition, digestion problems, and obsessive thinking about food. Although I've since conquered the need to starve myself after years of rebuilding my self-esteem, I'm still dealing with most of these anorexic symptoms.

My bout with anorexia is just one example of the driven personality that's so much a part of who I am. This drive is a powerful motivating tool, but also a destructive force. It can blind me to the harm I'm capable of inflicting on myself in my desire to prove I'm in control of my own life. I've juggled the pieces of my driven personality since early childhood, but my SCI experience has clearly amplified this trait tremendously.

I entered college with my self-esteem bruised but on the mend, with insecurities about body image and social judgment still tormenting my subconscious. I devoted myself to proving that I was different from other people with spinal cord injury, who seemed mainly interested in waiting for a cure that might never happen. I knew that if I wanted the world to notice me in a meaningful way, I would have to do something meaningful with my life. I wanted to leave my mark on the world, so I focused on a mission to change the way society saw people with disabilities. It gave me a sense of purpose and a reason to get up in the morning.

Despite my doubts, I embraced the positive side of my driven personality and focused on being successful. I suppose some would call it a coping mechanism. Paralysis generates a lot of powerful emotions for me, both positive and negative. Keeping myself busy and productive with writing, my studies, and being with friends prevented me from dwelling on what could have been. I pushed myself to challenge my limitations and explore my options every day. It made my life interesting, and making my life interesting was the critical key I used to unlock the chains of depression that initially imprisoned me after sustaining my injury.

In 1992, I graduated summa cum laude from Medaille College in Buffalo, New York, with a baccalaureate degree in media communications. I had the highest grade point average in my major and gave the commencement speech. That same year I won my community's Courage to Come Back Award, but it wasn't enough. I wanted to be celebrated for my talent, not my "bravery." My goal was to prove I was worthy of notice apart from my paralysis, not because of it.

My questions regarding sexuality continued to bother me throughout my early twenties. I had become curious but cautious after a few noncommittal kisses from male friends. A young woman I met in college with multiple sclerosis thought promiscuity meant popularity. The graphic descriptions she shared about her multiple sexual encounters repulsed me. I swore I would never allow myself to be used like that in a misguided quest to prove I was a woman. I had made a conscious decision to shelve my questions years earlier because I didn't like the answers I was getting from people with or without disabilities, and I hadn't been ready to find out through personal experimentation.

After moving out of Mom's house and into my first apartment at twenty-five, I met a wonderful man who taught me that intimacy was the greater part of intercourse. The mechanics of sex with paralysis were complicated, and my inexperience made for some challenging moments, but my fears that I was undesirable were alleviated in our laughter and shared exploration. I came to understand that sexuality was a product of self-esteem. Men were attracted to me when I felt attractive. The act itself is not as important as the sharing of our most intimate selves — although the act itself became darn fun once I learned to enjoy it!

In 1996, I accepted my first paying job as director of the Erie County Chapter of ThinkFirst National Traumatic Injury Prevention Programs, still forcing myself to ignore old insecurities when they tried to attack me with doubts in my newly acquired position. I'd finally gotten the chance to prove myself, and I was determined not to blow it. I began making a name for myself as the program earned national awards for excellence.

In 2001, the general manager of a local television station saw me speak at an event for the United Way. He approached me with a request to do some contributing reporting on ordinary people facing adversity with extraordinary strength. My first assignment was a piece about a local church support group for parishioners with disabilities. I went with my patented smile and the idea that I was helping them. I remember feeling much more comfortable with the cameraman than the group itself because I thought that he and I were on the same life level. We were career people doing our jobs. We weren't better. We were just different — or so I reasoned.

Then I stumbled upon a part of me that I never knew existed. I felt myself being drawn in by the group as I interviewed them individually. I began to see the mirror image of my own determination to be happy in each of their faces. I felt struck dumb, embarrassed by my own ego and horrified to realize that I'd been hiding from my own disability for years.

I went home that night and cried because the new reflection of quadriplegia in my mirror was so different from the image I had fostered for myself in my soul. It was time to accept the part of myself that I had been ignoring for so long. It brought me to a deeper, more honest sense of my own identity.

I was thirty-four years old before I finally found the balance of self-image, self-acceptance, and self-esteem that I needed to be happy. It took me twenty-two years to get here because it took that long to realize that I had been denying essential elements of who Kris Ann Piazza is. Once I let go of who I thought I should be, I was able to see who I am — and who I can be.

Living with a spinal cord injury as a grown woman is much different than I thought it would be as a young girl. My strong drive to succeed remains, but the energy that propels me is profoundly different, born more out of my inherently competitive personality than the fear of not measuring up to other's expectations. I'm no longer trying to prove myself in spite of my spinal cord injury.

My life is full and exciting instead of the misery I thought it would be when I was newly injured. I recently won the title of Ms. Wheelchair New York 2000, and today I'm the senior writer for a very large healthcare system and the proud author of a novel, *IMPACT*— a fictional story based on my life.

Now I think of the uncertain twelve-year-old girl who felt like nothing when she was THERE who has become something in the new millennium HERE, and I allow myself a little smile. There are no easy journeys after spinal cord injury, but people without disabilities often take just as long to find themselves. For me, the greatest difference between There and Here is a sense of self-worth.

I always had it. I just misplaced it for a while.

Kris Ann Piazza lives in Buffalo, New York. She works as the senior writer/editor for the largest health care system in Western New York and sits on various community boards. Kris is Ms. Wheelchair New York 2000, and is an accomplished traumatic injury prevention public speaker in her hometown.

SCI – My Path to Scientific Discovery

Sasha Rabchevsky

T5-6

Age at SCI: 19

Date of SCI: August 11, 1985

Lexington, Kentucky

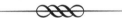

*I*n August, 1985 — just days before I was to begin my junior year at Hampden-Sydney College in Virginia and vie for a starting strong safety position on the football team — I became paralyzed from the chest down in a motorcycle accident. I was nineteen.

That moment would lead me to becoming an assistant professor in the Department of Physiology and Spinal Cord and Brain Injury Research Center at the University of Kentucky. Seventeen years ago, in the mountains of West Virginia, I never imagined my interests would turn to neuroscience research — or to loving life in Kentucky.

The last thing I remember was getting on the back of the motorcycle, without a helmet, huddled behind a childhood friend. The rescue crew lost my vital signs several times on the way to the hospital, where my parents were informed that I had fractured my fifth and sixth thoracic vertebrae. It was the first time they heard the word "paraplegic."

Numbed by the physician's words that I could be permanently

paralyzed, they asked, "But his legs have been moving since the accident, so how can he be paralyzed?" My mother had sworn she had seen me move my feet. This was likely function I had not yet lost to the continuing swelling and secondary damage to my spinal cord.

The best option for me was to be transferred was Georgetown University Hospital, where I faced complicated surgery and long-term rehabilitation. My first recollection was being shaved by a nurse telling me I had been in a coma for almost two weeks. Once she left me alone, I thought that I couldn't move my legs or arms because I was tied down. The moment was mixed with a morphine-induced, Alice In Wonderland-like hallucination, seemingly suspended above a record store aisle with endless slopes of albums on either side.

In truth, I was in a bed that slowly but continually rotated from side to side to relieve pressure on the sores on my backside. The emergency team had left me strapped onto a stretcher for more than fifteen hours, for fear of aggravating my other injuries. In his journal, my father wrote, "More than thirteen hours had passed and Sasha had not been moved from the stretcher, much less given an aspirin." He physically confronted a doctor, saying, "I'd rather my son die on an operating table than on that damn stretcher!"

Next, I remember a doctor telling me they implanted titanium rods to stabilize my spine but that my spinal cord was "clinically severed." He compared it to the broken bristles of a broom that remain intact, though permanently damaged. He gave me the old statistics spiel and said the potential for recovery was slim, saying that I might be able to drive a specially equipped van one day. I was soon in denial. I loved my Grand Prix. Why a van?! Anyway, how long before I get back to playing? Does the coach know I'll miss some games? Why are you saying I'm a "complete" paraplegic if my spinal cord is intact? Is a T5 injury better than a T6?

Initially, I really did want to take my life. At the time of my accident, I had reached the point where I was ready to leave the family home, and my parents were realizing and accepting it. Then I was suddenly more dependent than I had ever been. I couldn't accept being helped with things that used to be second nature — and personal. I refused anyone's help if I could still do it myself. My frustration mounted as therapists or loved ones pushed me. I wished I could implant all of my hopes, depression, fear, lack of sensation, and loss of mobility into everyone so they would understand the shit I was going through and just back off. I don't think my parents and sister realized how damn mad and guilty I felt for putting them through this.

It soon hit me that my whole life had changed — both a humbling experience and a kick in the ass I couldn't feel anymore. One morning toward the end of my stay at Georgetown, I remember feeling very warm and comfortable, despite all my fractures, and the room seemed luminescent even though it was early dawn. I woke my father, who was sleeping on a fold-out cot next to me, saying, "Pop, I'm okay. Everything's going to be okay."

To help cope with the transition, my mother and father attended SCI family support groups to learn as much as possible. In time, my parents and my sister began to accept that the initial shock was over, I was alive and getting better, and that overcoming this hurdle — while physically and emotionally exhausting — was not only possible but becoming a reality. My stubborn volition to do things for myself without assistance, if at all possible, had forced my parents to begin to accept my independence. Every increment of progress was a huge boost for everyone. Along with it came more self-confidence that I was not going to be a burden to my family. It also helped bring things back to a relatively normal state when my parents had to get back to their own lives.

The music of Bob Marley was a powerful inspiration during my recovery — the true messages behind his clouds of marijuana smoke. One particular quote became my mantra: "Every man thinks his burden is the heaviest." I saw the truth in these words through my rehab roommate, Stephen, a seventeen-year-old who was shot in the neck because he didn't have any money on him. How the hell do I complain about my day to a C5 quadriplegic who breathes through a tube in his throat, especially when he manages to smile every morning as we are woken by the "uprights?"

While others told me to have faith that I would walk again, I would say, "I don't give up hope, but I'm not holding my breath." Instead, I tried to help myself and others by focusing on the next step rather than on my mounting frustrations over my slow recovery or the complete lack of any treatments.

In rehab I tried to learn as much as possible about treatments for spinal cord injuries. Seeing that the prospects for recovery seemed dismal, I thought, "Why isn't there a cure?" If this damage is indeed irreparable, I want to be among the people declaring that. So I returned to rustic, inaccessible Hampden-Sydney a year later to reclaim my independence. I was able to graduate only a semester behind the rest of my class, and on to a graduate assistantship at the University of Florida to conduct spinal cord injury research.

Ten years after my accident, I earned a Ph.D. in Neuroscience and married Gisele Catherine Legare — who was willing to marry me, sell our house, ship our new car equipped with hand controls overseas, leave our pets with her folks, and move to Paris, France, all within a two-week period — where I did my first post-doctoral fellowship in neuroimmunology at the University of Paris.

We faced numerous challenges from the lack of awareness of disability issues in France. I never saw anyone else using a wheelchair, and I got many curious, unabashed stares. The teaching hospital I worked in was completely inaccessible, save for a "gerbil tube" connected to the medical school. Even though I had insisted in my contract that they provide accessible restrooms, parking, and that the tube would remain open while I was working, none of this had been done — until some medical students helped me power saw through the inaccessible bathroom stall doors.

Gisele and I met during a ride together to a beach house rented by a friend, instantly attracted to one another. She later told me she was intrigued about what I could and couldn't do — if you know what I mean. This speaks to Gisele's nature. She didn't care about my disability, she saw me for who I am and made me feel very comfortable. By the end of the long weekend our fate was sealed. We immediately began dating, and a year later I moved into her inaccessible house made accessible by her father. Gisele and I often reflect on the fact that we never would have met and been so happy together if I hadn't been paralyzed and she had not divorced her first husband. We have never felt our relationship is extraordinary, except that we love each other unequivocally.

After studying in Paris, I came back to the United States to work on potential spinal cord injury therapies at the University of Kentucky. Soon after receiving a state grant funded from speeding tickets and drunk-driving penalties, I was invited to the Kentucky state capitol when Christopher Reeve visited to help persuade the Kentucky legislature not to reallocate funds already committed to spinal cord research. A group of us from the university met with him in a round table format to answer questions about spinal cord injury and our research. I believe I was the first researcher he met who has a spinal cord injury. I wanted to speak in a way that supported his hopes, but convey that a cure in our lifetime is not a given — even with more research money. But he is driven by his personal cause and he continues to remind me of how much I still have — and must use.

Early in my rehabilitation, I made a vow to get my upper body as strong as possible, to get the muscles that still work to be as strong as possible. I came to accept that I would be using a wheelchair for a while, but I didn't believe it would be forever. One thing that really ate at me was the wasting away of my leg muscles. Therefore, I started to "walk" with crutches and leg braces, but it required assistance and was a bitch to do on a regular basis. I also tested a stationary bicycle system using functional electrical stimulation (FES) at the National Rehabilitation Hospital in Washington, D.C., where skin surface electrodes stimulated my legs. Weeks later my muscle mass increased, oxygen saturation levels and consumption rates improved, meaning that my body (engine) was utilizing energy (gas) more efficiently, like an athlete in training.

More than ten years later, I enrolled in a program here at the University of Kentucky, in collaboration with the Cleveland FES Center. In January 2002 surgeons placed eight electrodes deep in the muscles of my lower back, buttocks, and upper legs. The thirteen surgical cuts included a seven-inch slice in my abdomen that holds the system's stimulator that enables me to stand up with a walker and ambulate — albeit with strenuous effort, and a gait akin to Frankenstein's monster. My decision was based on personal desire mixed with a motive for scientific investigation mixed with meeting the right people.

The recovery was the longest three months of my life, and I wondered if I should have gone through the surgery. Then, in April I stood up in parallel bars for the first time, "Houston, we have stand-up!" In October I stood and "walked" across the stage to give the keynote address at an international neurotrauma symposium. My message to that scientific audience — and to any skeptics who question the procedure — was that, "I chose this radical procedure to improve the quality of my life." Such that I can stand up and kiss Gisele. For therapeutic purposes, of course!

With my years of research experience, I have no illusions about the huge scientific obstacles in front of me and other scientists. But fifteen years after my accident, promoting regeneration in the injured spinal cord is now a reality. We still face the challenge of directing damaged nerve fibers to the desired targets for functional recovery. Ultimately, successful treatments will involve a combination of therapies. There will be no magic bullet. Moreover, going from paralysis to full control of motion may be overly optimistic — walking is a tall order.

Once therapies do evolve, we will be like babies learning to walk all over again, but with a fundamentally different neural circuitry. What lost function do you wish to recover most? How about two or three levels of sensation back? I say to anyone hoping for a cure — do everything to increase the probability that such therapies will work by staying in the best physical condition possible.

In the scientific arena, I see the good, the bad, and the ugly on a daily basis. Despite my apparent scientific skepticism, this is a decisive era in research, so I keep working on a treatment. While I may not benefit from my own research, I hope it will eventually help others with spinal cord injury.

Alexander "Sasha" Rabchevsky is an assistant professor of physiology at the University of Kentucky, where his current research focus is seeking a treatment for autonomic dysreflexia, a potentially life-threatening complication with some spinal cord injuries, which he experiences himself on a daily basis. He and his wife enjoy the company of two dogs and three cats, doing outdoor activities in the hills of Kentucky and working out together at the gym.

Growing Through Adversity

Flo Kahn
C5-6
Age at SCI: 35
Date of SCI: June 8, 1973
Northfield, Minnesota

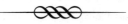

*T*wenty-nine years ago, I broke my neck. I was thirty-five years old, married, expecting my first child, and living a full and busy life as wife, pediatric nurse, and semi-professional singer. On my way home from work, I was sitting at a stoplight when I was rear-ended.

I woke up in the emergency room as they were putting Crutchfield tongs in my head and said, "There goes my life." While the nurse in me sensed physical paralysis, my statement had many layers reflecting the many other parts that made up who I was.

I was now a C5-6 quad with complete motor paralysis from the chest down and an incomplete sensory injury that caused me to feel a buzzing sensation below the level of injury. I was placed on a Stryker frame and turned every two hours. After a spinal fusion was done, I developed adult respiratory distress syndrome that necessitated getting a tracheotomy and being on a respirator for weeks. The high oxygen blew a hole from my trachea into my esophagus.

When I was in respiratory intensive care dealing with survival, the rehabilitation team still came and put my hands in night splints. Getting to rehab seemed unattainable. Through good medical care and breaking down big hurdles into small pieces, I got off the respirator. I still kept the tracheotomy. That problem would be faced later.

I was in shock. My feelings remained frozen inside. If I had felt all the losses, I might have exploded. I felt like a spectator watching all the things done to my body. After going on the respirator, labor started and my baby girl was born. She lived three days. My mother insisted I be told even though I was unconscious. She played a tape of me singing Bach's "Lord, have mercy on me." I cried and was told about Kristina's birth and death. Although I mouthed that I wanted her cremated and buried between my grandparents, I have no recollection of this. If something is broken into enough small pieces, a person *can* participate, and grieve. So much had been ripped away, I felt hopeless.

My husband and mother stayed close. Since my father recently had two heart attacks, giving emotional support initially was just too stressful for him. My four siblings were busy with their lives and families and felt heartsick and helpless.

When I finally got off the respirator, I was excited to be moving to rehab. I went to PT and OT twice every day and had to re-learn how to do the simplest skills. I felt ashamed. I was like a little baby going back to early achievements. Everything I had been able to do with my body was gone, and I felt like I was gone too. My OT helped me feel better about myself by arranging to have my hair cut and tipped and teaching me how put in my contact lenses.

Getting beyond these everyday tasks to a life with meaning and purpose meant coping and getting all of me back together. This happened like putting puzzle pieces back together. As I worked on physical tasks those first months, my emotions moved through different stages.

I had learned about stages of grieving in nursing. There is no time frame for grieving; each person has his/her own journey. The first stage is impact — the time of shock when feelings are closed out to protect the person. The head knows what's happening, but not the heart. The second stage is disruption — the reality of losses emerge with feelings of sadness, fear, anger, and guilt. The third stage is recovery/restructuring — feelings are less intense and new skills and roles begin. At any time, intense feelings can be triggered bringing a person back to disruption. The last stage is growth — you can talk about your losses, feel good about feeling better, reinvest in life, and find new balance.

Initially, I was in shock, but disruption and recovery popped in and out. At first, I went to therapies like a robot, feeling shame at learning simple skills again. There was disruption when I got mad because I wasn't asked how I thought I was doing. There was more disruption when I saw my first wheelchair and the claw-like splint that gives me the ability to pinch — I cried. I was eager to get home, denying the loss of all the activities that I couldn't do! Going through these emotional stages was like an endless dance — going back and forth for years.

Home was filled with what I formerly did. Being unable to take care of the house frustrated me. Having no finger movement to knit, play piano, sculpt, or cook made me deeply sad. Not being able to make love as before made me feel guilty and inadequate. As these feelings finally began to surface, I coped by being stoic and pushing them away — as I had learned growing up in a family of Norwegian-German heritage. I know now that it took lots of energy to keep feelings inside. I became very depressed, spending days doing nothing, with no clue what to do. My brain may have known about grieving, but I had never grieved.

I stayed depressed for five years while dealing with continuing lung problems. Once, when I was at Sister Kenny Rehab with a lung infection, the psychologist told me I was depressed. I looked at her dumbfounded. Well ... yeah!!! But no action was taken by the psychologist or me. I wonder if being a nursing professional slowed people in helping me. I might have gotten help sooner if someone had said, "You're depressed because you are dealing with many losses. Talking about your losses will help."

My husband wanted his Flo back. He helped by finding a surgeon in Boston for a successful tracheo-esophageal fistula repair, and then sending me to Craig Rehab. With new energy from the successful surgery, I worked on more physical skills. With Craig's excellent classes and educational materials, I took more responsibility for my body by learning how to teach others about it. Yet, I felt defeat and more shame when I couldn't do C5-6 skill expectations like moving my body across the mats or emptying my leg bag because of my long torso and short arms.

When I got home, I was able to make decisions about how to utilize my time and energy better. However, I wasn't back in balance yet. When my husband suggested attending the local spinal cord injury group, I said no — that meant being with people who were disabled!

Although adjusting in some areas, I remained depressed. My husband was discouraged and having trouble with our relationship. He suggested that I go to Courage Center, a new transitional rehab facility nearby. Since the clients at Courage are placed in the managerial role of living independently, I led weekly team meetings of my rehab team to keep track of my goals. My life was busy and enjoyable — living and interacting with others with disabilities. We all got to know one another as people.

While at Courage, I was stunned to learn that my oldest brother's wife had committed suicide, and that my husband wanted a divorce! My dam of stoicism broke. With a good counselor helping me, I finally began to deal with all the losses. Each week I talked and cried about what I'd lost — my hands, my standing self, my singing voice, my baby, my marriage, on and on. Each session was like boulders on a beach. I'd deal with the boulders — losses — and the next week more would surface. As my buried feelings emerged, I realized I was still me — a whole and valuable person. I wasn't just working hands or a singing voice. Although I valued those parts of me, I experienced a deeper sense of knowing myself. Grieving was hard work and took a year — my growth was well worth it.

All the pieces were coming together. Counseling freed up my energy and supported my returning self-esteem. Taking control of my care prepared me for independent living as did learning new daily living skills — eating, writing, typing.

As I recovered, I became involved in the resident council and peer counseling training. Then, the volunteer director asked me to be a tour guide for the center. I declined, thinking I should be doing some big nursing job. Finally, I gave in. This was a good step because I was using my brain again with the public and experienced increasing confidence. More opportunities opened up for me. It just took starting.

Before I left Courage, a new volunteer director noticed I seemed depressed, but heard about my education and saw potential. She asked me to help train new community volunteers and share my story with them. Through these trainings, I grew at a deeper level. Putting my experiences into words really helped me communicate that while all of me was affected by my disability, the disability was just a part of me.

Doing the trainings, I realized that society's stereotypes about people with disabilities were also in me. When going to a class once, I saw a man with cerebral palsy going inside too. I thought, "Oh, there's day care for the retarded here." When I entered my classroom, he was setting up a projector. "Oh, he's the video technician." He was the teacher!!

The thought of having a disability is scary to adults. Seeing only the paralyzed body, they believe: can't walk, talk, think, work, or marry. People also fear saying the "wrong thing" — about things they think we can't do. At trainings, I explained that people with SCI are interested in many things and that it is okay to talk about anything — I have a disability, but my life and my interests are not any different from those of people without SCI.

Because the trainings were successful, I was given the responsibility of leading the groups through the entire attitude awareness training process. While busy with the trainings, I moved into my own apartment. I was ready to start living — not just existing. I advertised for attendants, and hired and trained them. Over time, working and living with attendants, I learned about communication, conflict resolution, and living with different personality types. Good attendant support brought stability at home and enabled me to move into a seventeen-year career of speaking, training, and nursing education — until I retired. My life had become meaningful and more balanced — including having fun and being involved socially in the community.

The spiritual part of me emerged when I was asked to speak in churches during the International Year of the Disabled. I grew up as a Lutheran and had never shared my faith with others. My live-in attendant came with me to one church and listened as a man asked me how I had grown spiritually. I got stuck trying to answer. I realized that my spiritual space was filled with an intellectual understanding of my faith that was challenged by my injury. I grappled with the relevance of my faith as my live-in attendant kept questioning me. As she questioned me, I got angry, but grew spiritually through this dialogue. So much of me had changed with this accident, did my faith have to change too? I had been stuck — not realizing I was on a journey. Suffering propelled growth and renewed my faith. It was no longer just intellectual; my journey was heartfelt. I was further nurtured when I joined a church family, went to Bible study groups, and grew closer in my personal relationship with Christ.

My accident threw all of me into chaos — intellectually, emotionally, and spiritually. I was more paralyzed emotionally and spiritually than physically! These parts of me came back together thanks to the people who helped me grieve, learn new skills, examine my beliefs, and discover new opportunities.

The love and prayers of my family and friends supported me in discovering that I wasn't just a body — what it could or couldn't do — and that I could live a full life from a wheelchair!

I live each day knowing I am valuable and worthwhile as a whole person with much to give — and learn.

Florence Stroebel Kahn lives in Northfield, Minnesota. She enjoyed many years teaching nurses about SCI and training the public on attitude awareness. Currently, she lives in a log home and enjoys painting, nature study, music, family genealogy, and helping in church ministries.

Coming Full Circle

Kris Gulden
T4
Age at SCI: 31
Date of SCI: May 26, 1998
Centreville, Virginia

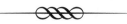

O n May 26, 1998, after Shamu, my yellow Lab, and I drove home from Pennsylvania, I went out for a ride on my bike. Within twenty minutes of home, a car hit me from behind. I sustained a bruised and displaced spinal cord at the T4 level and a traumatic brain injury. I also broke four vertebrae, two ribs, my breastbone, my right clavicle and a tooth, and had lots of cuts that required stitches or staples.

I spent ten days in Fairfax (Virginia) Hospital and gradually started to understand what had happened. Since I had no recollection of the accident, my Dad explained why I was in the hospital. When I was transferred to the rehab hospital, I still had no idea how severely I'd been injured. Although I'd been told that I had about a twenty percent chance of ever walking again, it didn't sink in.

I was at Mount Vernon Rehabilitation Hospital for two months. Despite many hours of physical and occupational therapy, and the services of doctors, nurses, the social worker, and the neuropsychologist, nothing prepared me for what it would really be like to live with a spinal cord injury. I don't think anybody could have explained how drastically my life would change.

Prior to the accident, I heavily identified with my job and my hobbies. I was a police officer and a triathlete. I loved working the midnight patrol shift. When I wasn't working, I was either on my bike, running, swimming, or working out at the gym. If I wasn't competing, I was training.

In the first months after the accident, thinking about my future, I envisioned myself maintaining the same relationships with the same people. While my career and some of my hobbies would change, I expected to travel around the country and compete. Instead of triathlons, I would compete in the wheelchair division of marathons — only my means of transportation would change. But that vision was not realistic because my needs had changed. In public, I had to be concerned about accessibility and factor bathroom issues into the equation. And I was dealing with physical pain that, at times, kept me home in bed.

As my discharge from the hospital drew near, I was filled with excitement and fear. I couldn't wait to get back to my own house. I missed Shamu and my own surroundings. But I had grown accustomed to trained nurses providing for my medical needs and was nervous about returning to my condo — with my mother as my primary caretaker. I had no idea how we would get along as room-mates, and I was apprehensive about my personal care because my mom has very limited strength in her hands from rheumatoid arthritis. I was still unable to transfer without assistance, and I wasn't sure Mom could help. And since I had only tried the bowel program a few times in the hospital, I was unsure how we would accomplish it.

Within days, Mom and I learned how healing laughter can be. One night, we were preparing for the bowel program when disaster struck. It would have been absolutely humiliating under any other circumstances. But for a newly injured paraplegic and her untrained, unpaid, attendant mom, there was nothing to do but laugh. In that moment, our relationship changed more than I ever thought it would. And, we learned the most important tool for coping — our senses of humor.

After discharge, I learned that Kaiser Permanente, my HMO, was refus-ing to pay my medical bills. Although I'd never been interested in politics and led a fairly nondescript life in the suburbs of Washington, D.C., I became more recognizable for two reasons. In September, a group of friends began working on a 5K road race to raise money for my ongoing medical expenses and to raise awareness about SCI. Then in October, thanks to the public information officer at the police department, the *Washington Post* did a human interest story about me. In May 1999, the first Annual May Day 5K race was held. Overall, my first year post-injury was a blur. In November, I returned to work on a part-time basis, and was lifting weights and riding the recumbent bicycle at the gym. By Christmas, I was able to walk with the rolling walker. My recovery and my battle with Kaiser distracted me from seeing how much my life had changed.

Because I thought that I would enjoy continued recovery of function, I pushed myself to stick with a stringent rehab program. Since I was still ambulatory, my sense of self had not changed as drastically as if I'd been completely reliant on my chair. I was still able to walk into the gym, around the office, through stores, and when I went out with friends. But in September 1999, I noticed that my left hand was weakening. In November, a myelogram caused me to lose almost total use of my left hand. Later, I learned that a syrinx (a post-traumatic cyst, or fluid-filled cavity) was putting pressure on my spinal cord. The only solution was to operate. Between Christmas 1999 and April 2000, I had seven operations and another myelogram, spent another month in the rehab hospital, and retired from my job. I had the hardest time accepting the fact that I lost total use of my legs and bladder after the second operation.

Five years have passed since my accident, and I'm still adjusting. Actually, including the operations, I've had multiple spinal cord injuries. If there had been only one incident, who knows how I'd be getting around now?

Shortly after my accident, I knew that I would never be a police officer again. I also knew that I would never find a job I loved as much. Today, I still don't know what I want to do with the rest of my life. At times, I feel inadequate when I compare myself to other people with SCI who seem to be doing so much — going to law school, raising children, working full time jobs. I have to remind myself that each of us is on an individual journey — I am okay the way I am. I have changed "inferior" to "inadequate" in Eleanor Roosevelt's "nobody can make you feel inferior without your consent" and adopted it as my new outlook.

I am still capable of making valuable contributions to the world.

In January 2002, after reading about the Quest for the Cure program at Rutgers University, I called for information and had a lengthy conversation with a staff person. In February, I received a call from a woman who was scheduled to testify on behalf of the Coalition for the Advancement of Medical Research (CAMR) before the Senate Judiciary Committee in Washington. Since she was sick, she called the person at Rutgers for help in finding someone to speak at the hearing and was referred to me. With less than a week's notice, I testified on behalf of CAMR. I was so nervous. I felt like the hopes and dreams of millions were resting on my shoulders. When the hearing was over, I knew that I had come through — and opened doors for myself. The two people from the Christopher Reeve Paralysis Foundation, who had helped me through my testimony, said that they often needed people to speak because Christopher Reeve can't be everywhere. I was being asked to fill in for Superman!

Since then, I have spoken about therapeutic cloning in California, recorded a public service radio advertisement for CAMR, spoken to media representatives as a patient advocate, and spoken at press conferences and hearings. It has been incredibly gratifying and empowering to play a role in government and to realize that I have talents and gifts that can help people.

I was thirty-one years old when I was injured. Eighteen months later, I had become much closer to my mother. Because I wanted to be honest with her about who I am, I told my family and my closest friends my secret of twenty years — I am gay. The news was well received by all. More importantly, sharing that part of my life has been very freeing.

Looking back at the last five years, I'm surprised that so much time has passed. The physical adjustment to living with a spinal cord injury seems to have taken place naturally, with little thought or effort. For example, the first few times I took my chair apart to put it in my car, I wondered if it would always be that much work. Yet I knew that the more I did it, the easier it would become. This has been true of every physical task from transferring onto the tub bench to putting electrodes on my legs and hooking up the cables to ride my StimMaster bike.

Emotional adjustment has been much more difficult. I never realized how isolated and dependent on others I would become, how much exertion is required just to keep up with my friends, or how much planning and preparation is necessary to get through each day. One of the biggest challenges has been "accepting" my injury because to me, "accepting" means giving up. I hate when the word "disabled" is used to describe me because I don't think it does. I believe that I have the ability to change my situation, and I work hard to do so. I believe that my paralysis is temporary, and that I will walk again. Yet, to survive and function, I live with a level of acceptance.

Until that day comes, I can choose to make concessions in order to enjoy myself. For example, when I travel, I need to be able to use the bathroom on an airplane. I've decided that it suits me better to ask a stranger to help me pull my pants up than not travel.

Until I started working part-time recently, I missed interacting with people. I tried to get out each day — to meet a friend or volunteer somewhere. I've learned that good friends are willing to help. When my friends invite me out, even though they may have to push my chair, help me over curbs, through doors, or up steps, they want me to be there.

My sense of worth was once tied to the medals and trophies I had won. I have shoeboxes full of ribbons and plaques, and a scrapbook with newspaper clippings reporting how fast I could swim. Now, I ride a stationary bike that uses electrical stimulation to move my legs. I am capable of riding sixteen miles, though I don't move an inch. In this stillness, I am finding my true mettle. And, while I spend the majority of my time sitting, I feel like I've become a much taller person.

One of the most interesting changes is my shift in focus from criminal justice to social justice. I can still influence lives by being a mentor to young girls through the Girls In Training program, speaking at high school assemblies during disability awareness month, or testifying before the Senate. My sense of satisfaction now comes from feeling that I'm making a difference in the lives of others.

In June 2003, one month after the Fifth Annual May Day 5K race, I bought a handcycle. With my handcycle, I can ride and exercise outside again — and compete in races again. In October 2003, I will compete in the Marine

Corps Marathon. I have come full circle!

In some ways, I was right when I thought that only my means of transportation would change. I am the same person — residing in a different body. My injury has given me a chance to acknowledge and accept who I really am. Initially, I told people that the accident cut to the core of me. Although it did, it has not changed the core of me. At first, I thought that the inability to catch burglars and run eight-minute miles had radically altered who I am. I see now that is not true.

Kris Gulden lives in Centreville, Virginia. She is a sales specialist at REI and looks forward to racing in her handcycle. While working on this essay, Kris lost her companion of twelve years, Shamu.

My Bag of Tools

Larry Nitz
T12
Age at SCI: 35
Date of SCI: May 2, 1983
Havre, Montana

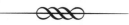

O n May 2, 1983, I became paraplegic. I remember the day vividly — a sunny, fairly warm but windy spring day. I was working as an electric lineman in north central Montana, less than a mile from where I worked for a pig farmer when I was in high school. I was happy to be alive and feeling lucky to have a job where I was able to work outdoors. I loved my job, was proud of my profession, and proud of the company I worked for.

I remember an incredible stab of pain when I grazed an ungrounded conductor with my shoulder. It was common practice to climb through these lines, unprotected, because they were usually grounded, since they were no longer in use. Not this one. As I was falling, I thought that it was no big deal. I would just get up, dust myself off, and climb back up the pole. But then the pain when I landed was the most intense pain I'd ever experienced in my life. The fall broke my back at T12 and L1. It also broke my right wrist. I passed in and out of consciousness. I remember hearing one of my coworkers calling mayday on the two-way radio.

I saw a woman kneeling over me and wondered if she was an angel. I asked her who she was. She said, "My name is Lois. Is it alright if I pray for you?" The pain became a little more bearable as she started praying.

Several years ago, after two and a half months in the hospital and in rehab — and a lot of living — I was seeing a counselor, who asked me to write a letter to my injury, describing my anger. I thought, "Well this won't take long, because I'm not angry." A strange thought since I was seeing the counselor because my wife had moved out of the house. I knew I had to get serious about making some changes in my confrontational behavior if I wanted to get her back.

Three long, tear-filled days later I finished the letter. I never realized how angry I was. For some reason, this letter helped me purge my anger. I'm not angry anymore. In fact, I think I'm happier now than I've ever been in my entire life.

Damn You!
You took away my identity. You took away my reason to be a man.
Damn You!
You took away the work I loved. When I was "in the hooks" I always looked forward to getting up in the morning and going to work. I loved the smell of the wood and the leather, the feel of the hooks on my feet, and the creaking sounds the pole made. I miss the perspective of the world from the top of a pole. I miss the camaraderie of my coworkers. I wish I hadn't sold my tools after my injury. I thought I had to sell them when I came home from the hospital. They were a part of me, a part of my identity. I always took good care of my tools and I was proud of them. Now I miss them and want them back.
Damn You!
Do you know I have to work indoors now, at a desk, and put up with office politics and bosses who don't understand what it means to work outside and then be forced to stop what you love doing? I could be outside, away from all that aggravation if it wasn't for you.
Damn You!
Do you know it takes me two hours every day just to have a bowel

movement? I sit on the throne and stick my finger up my ass for two hours just so I don't get sick or crap my pants.

Damn You!

You took away my sexuality. Do you know I can't feel my penis? I forgot what it feels like to have a "normal" orgasm like a "normal" man. Do you know how frustrating that is?

Damn You!

Do you know I can't even pee like a "normal" man? I have to insert a plastic tube up my penis to drain my bladder. Do you know I get bladder infections all the time? Do you know a bladder infection has the potential to kill me?

Damn You!

Do you know I can't even turn over in bed without sitting up? I have to wake up and turn over so I don't get pressure sores. I would love to be able to sleep through the night without waking up six or seven times.

Damn You!

Do you know that some nights I don't sleep because of the pain I'm in from over-using my shoulders and hands? Do you know I had to give up playing wheelchair basketball because my joints couldn't take it anymore?

Damn You!

I watch my wife do things that no woman should have to do. Things that I used to do, but now she has to, because I'm not able. This injury has taken a toll on her body as well.

Damn You!

Do you know that some people look at me with disdain and disgust? Do you know I feel discriminated against because of my disability? Do you know I've seen parents pull their children away when they try to approach me?

Damn You!

Do you know I can't even feel if I hurt myself, or if I get too cold or too hot? I have burned my feet and don't even know how it occurred. Do you know that it's hours after I go to bed in the winter time before my feet get warm?

Thank You!

You made me realize how important and precious life is and not to take it for granted. You made me take a long, hard look at the way I lived my life and made me realize I needed to make some big changes in my priorities.

Thank You!

You probably made me a better lover to my mate because I'm not able to have a "normal" orgasm. I take more time and pay more attention to her needs while making love. You made me realize that there is more to making love than having sex.

Thank You!

My life as a paraplegic seems "normal" now. My bowel program is just part of my everyday routine. It's not always convenient, but I try to make good use of the time as my own private time. I even have a TV and VCR in my bathroom so I can watch TV if I choose.

Thank You!

As a result of you, I was able to participate in wheelchair sports for a time. I really regret not participating in sports in high school. In a small way, I was able to relive my childhood through wheelchair sports, and that felt good!

Thank You!

As a result of my disability, and not being out of town working, I was able to be a larger part of my children's school life and extracurricular activities while they were growing up. I believe they are more loving, caring, and tolerant because of their experiences with me and my disability.

Thank You!

I'm more and more comfortable with myself and my disability. I believe I'm a better person because of my disability, because of the way it has forced me to adjust to different situations, and the way I live my life. I think I'm more patient, more tolerant, and more understanding of other people. I'm more compassionate, and more able to relate to people of differing abilities and from different walks of life.

Thank You!

You made me look at the world from the eyes of a person with a disability and realize that things were not going to change unless we, the disability community, take the time and invest the effort to effect that change. I'm proud to have made a difference. I'll never stop advocating for the people in this world who tend to slip through the cracks.

Thank You!

I'm retired now, and it's a rare occasion when Linda (my wife) and I are apart for more than a couple hours. I love my life! I love Linda more than life itself. I love spending time with my grandkids, and they enjoy me. We have a hotrod pickup and cruise in it on any given summer evening. I love traveling around the area in our trailer every summer. I enjoy shooting sports (especially cowboy action shooting) and although I'm not able to push a manual wheelchair through rough terrain anymore, I recently purchased a power chair for such activities. I enjoy woodworking and my skills as a woodworker have blossomed since I've been retired.

Thank You!

For teaching us that life goes on. It isn't always wonderful, but the alternative is worse. Linda has had to make adjustments, too. She had knee replacement surgery last year and will probably have the other one replaced soon. She also has arthritis in her back. These are small things in our eyes. Making adjustments as we age is a necessity for able-bodied and disabled alike. Linda and I are both happy — we have each other and that is the most important thing.

Thank You!

I really believe there is a God, who actually cares about us and looks over us. I think He has helped me arrive at this point in my life. I don't think I could have become the person I am today if I had not become paraplegic.

Epilogue

A few years ago I was a judge at the Linemans' Rodeo at Holter Dam in Montana. As I was going back to our motorhome having just finished judging my events, a young man stepped in front of me and asked, "Do you know who I am?"

"No, I can't say that I do," I said.

He introduced himself as the fellow that I had sold my tools to after my injury. I said, "No kiddin'! You still have 'em?"

"I sure do," he answered "In fact, I competed with them this morning.

Would you like to take a look at them?"

I said, "I sure would!," And with that, he led the way to his pickup where he reached into the back and pulled out a tool belt. I could tell without a doubt they were my old tools — some repairs I had made on them were still visible.

He said, "Would you like to have them back?"

I said, "I sure would, how much do you want for them?"

"Nothing," he said. "They're yours."

I could hardly hold back the tears as I hurried back to the motor home to show Linda. We hugged each other and cried like babies. This young man later told me that he knew the day I sold the tools to him that someday I would want them back. In fact, he told me that he had looked for me at the rodeo the year before — before I wrote my letter to my injury. But I wouldn't have been ready for his gift. I didn't know yet how much those tools meant to me.

After visiting with the fellow and his wife, we found out that he had worked in Montana for a couple of years, then moved to California for about six years. He then moved to Washington State and worked for a few more years, before finding a steady job and moving back to Montana. My tools had worked in three states, taught numerous apprentices the trade, and still found their way home.

I plan to make a shadow box or case of some kind out of old cedar power poles to display these wonderful artifacts. Someday I'll show them to my grandchildren and tell them the story of my lost tools. Miracles do happen. Linda and I pray that a magical and wonderful thing like this lightens your load in life too.

I feel like the luckiest person in the world.

Larry Nitz and his wife of thirty-five years, Linda, live in Havre, Montana, having raised two sons who have given them three grandchildren — who he lists among his favorite hobbies. Others are woodworking, camping, cowboy action shooting, and hot rods. He is involved with independent living locally and statewide, and is a local affiliate for the Rocky Mountain Region ADA Technical Assistance Center.

Devil's Night

Audrey Begay
C4-5
Age at SCI: 25
Date of SCI: October 31, 1997
Lakewood, Colorado

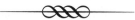

T wo weeks before my injury, while I was living in Durango, Colorado, my younger brother and I were sitting at a red light when we saw a young woman in a wheelchair pushing herself across the street in front of us. We both said, "I'd hate to be like that." I went on, "If I ever end up like that, I want you to kill me. Okay? No matter what." My brother nodded and asked the same of me. The light turned green and we sped past the woman as we talked about how hard it must be to have to use a wheelchair. I soon found out for myself.

On a cold Halloween night, 1997, I had attended a costume contest with my sister and brother-in-law dressed as Frankenstein's bride. Just before midnight, when we returned home, my sister and I had an argument. She got up and left the house. I felt bad and ran out the front door wearing dress shoes that didn't go well with ice. I slipped and landed on my neck. I lay there dazed.

My sister had no idea what had just happened and drove off thinking I was okay. I looked up at the dark sky as snow started to float down and couldn't understand what was going on. I tried to yell and scream, but only a whisper came out. My arms rested on my chest as my hands curled in. I finally drifted off into sleep. Fortunately, my brother woke up several hours later. He didn't see me until he opened the front door to let my dogs in. He quickly called 911, and I was whisked away as Frankie's bride.

I was diagnosed a C4-5 quadriplegic — paralyzed from the neck down. I was placed on a ventilator to help me breathe because my lungs and my diaphragm had collapsed. My vocal cords were partially paralyzed — that's why I couldn't yell. Then, they placed a halo on my head and screwed four bolts into my skull to hold it in place. They tightened it every week. I couldn't have a shower until it came off — four long months later.

Everything had changed for my family and me. It was hell! I kept re-running the thought of my last able-bodied day over and over in my head. My family got together and had to take charge of my life and make decisions for me because I was not able to communicate, and the doctors didn't think I'd make it through the first night. My family was overcome with the reality of the situation and cried. I heard their tears and sorrow. It was a very grim day.

After a few weeks in a coma, I woke up and felt scared. But, as long as my fiancé was there, I believed that I could face anything. We were to be married on Valentine's Day. Soon, I went to start my new life at Craig Hospital in Denver.

As the Christmas/New Year holidays approached, my family and I were depressed because of where we were. Then, on Valentine's Day, my fiancé dumped me. I was devastated. It broke my heart when he said, "This is so unattractive," as he kicked the tires on my wheelchair. He went on to say, "I'm young and want to travel and ride my bike or ski." I could see the disgust in his eyes as he brought up feeling weird if we were to ever have sex again. I begged him not to leave and reminded him about his promise to stick by my side no matter what and that he had said he loved me unconditionally. Bull crap! His eyes were cold and he walked out of my life with no remorse.

I was so hurt by his rejection — it felt harder to accept than my paralysis. Living this new life was going to be hard to accept if I was going to be abandoned by important people in my life. I hit bottom. I didn't eat or speak for two weeks. Being rejected by someone who I thought loved me was unbearable. I just kept crying — through the days and nights. It was a very depressing time. Yet, I realized that I had to continue my life. I had encouragement from my family and everyone at Craig. When they helped me see that others had it worse then I did, I started to try to make an effort.

My family was my backbone. They weren't going to let me give up. Because money was tight and the road trips to Denver were tiring everyone out, my family decided to relocate two of my brothers, Louis and Arthur, to Denver. Louis helped me stay focused on my recovery, and Arthur was the breadwinner. This was tough because we all had to pinch pennies. But, with the support of Louis and Arthur, we all made it through. Their support was all I needed. I felt that I had to make it for us.

It was rough the first year. I started to regain more movement as I pushed myself to be independent. I was tired of asking for help and took chances on any new task. I felt great when I could do simple things like brushing my teeth or feeding myself. I knew I had to try. It was a wonderful feeling to know that I could still do things for myself.

I felt a little more human and started keeping a journal to practice my writing and release my frustrations — not being able to scratch my nose, empty my urine bag, or put on my make-up. My brothers were always there to encourage me.

After five months at Craig, I moved in with my brothers. But living in close quarters became difficult, and I decided that I needed my own place. I applied for housing through the Section 8 Voucher Program and was accepted. The program pays about eighty percent of the rent; I pay the difference. I found a condo in a wonderful neighborhood.

The major adjustment for me was learning to depend on others. At first, six years ago, I got annoyed when my aides did simple tasks differently from me and at their own pace. I like things done quickly and thoroughly. Since then, I've had to allow strangers — including some drug addicts, drunks, thieves, and liars — into my home. It has been very hard to find good, honest, normal, and reliable aides. Fortunately, I finally found two good aides for now (knock on wood).

Everyone encouraged me to start dating, and my aides arranged some blind dates. Initially, I felt nervous and insecure about guys seeing me spasm or needing my urine bag emptied. As it turned out, the guys I dated never gave a thought to my chair. They saw Audrey, not the pain in the ass chair. I never sensed that the extra headache of transfers in and out of the car or the breakdown of my electric wheelchair bothered them. However, I never asked for assistance with my drainage bag and tried to control my spasms.

During this time, I met a nice fellow who worked as a technician at Craig. At first, we were strictly acquaintances. Much later, Adrian and I started to date. I felt so comfortable with him. I was in no hurry to jump into a relationship. Or so I thought. Six months later, we moved in together.

Two years later, I was pregnant. My family, friends, and doctors were scared. But, I was confident about my pregnancy because I thought I was quite healthy and in perfect shape to have a baby. But, being pregnant was hard on my body. Beginning in the third month, my spasms increased. Morning sickness came with full force, and I developed a bad bladder infection that landed me in the E.R. As the baby got bigger, I had to cut down being in my chair and I hyper-reflexed more then usual. In the last month, I was on bed rest.

It was all worth it! Adrian and I got through the nine months. Hannah, our beautiful baby girl, was born on Valentine's Day, 2000. I had no complications. Adrian and I have now been together for five years.

As a new mother, I had to take on more than I thought I could handle. I only have my right hand with some finger movement to work with. I was nervous about being left alone with Hannah. But, I didn't have anyone to help me take care of her. I bit the bullet and took on the challenge. Every day there was something new for me to tackle or improvise — preparing her bottles with hot tap water or changing her diapers with one hand. Thank God for Velcro diapers — a quad's best friend! Now she's three, and there are still new situations for both of us, like taking her to the park alone and hoping she won't fall. I like getting to help the other kids understand about disabilities by answering their questions.

Being in a wheelchair isn't easy. I need to worry about my intake of water, how long I'm up in my chair (to prevent sores), bladder infections, weight shifts, staying on a healthy diet, and avoiding accidents (who could love their bowel program?). I also need to deal with constant changes in my routine whenever I have to find a new aide. But, I don't sit around and cry about feeling miserable. Instead, I try to make life easier by getting physical therapy, going out with family or friends, getting more education to start a career, or writing my autobiography.

I struggle sometimes living with my harsh reality. I have to make sacrifices because I have a child to care for. I don't have the luxury of deciding to give up. I was once completely paralyzed from my neck down but I have worked my ass off to be able to improve my abilities.

Sadly, I've lost many friends and my fiancé. I even lost my best friend because she was jealous of me because I got so much attention. It has certainly been hurtful to be rejected, treated like damaged goods, and abandoned. But, I also have lots of new friends who admire me a great deal. I don't let my defenses down as easily as I used to because I'm tired of getting screwed over or lied to.

My injury helped me face issues within myself as well as my past. I was raised in a very abusive home. Looking back, I realize that I ran from city to city to drown out the memories. Then, when my relationship with my first love ended and I didn't know where to go, I returned home to Durango. There I led a lonely life. It was extremely depressing and I didn't think that it could get any worse. I was very vulnerable and rebounded into the engagement that ended after my injury. In Durango, I also saw all the animosity that my siblings had toward each other from incidents that occurred when we were children.

A few years after my injury, I dealt with our family issues and our past by speaking to every sibling alone, one after another. I apologized for all of my wrongdoing. By confronting the skeletons in my closet with my family, I started to feel like a whole new person and knew that I needed to change in order to make a better life for myself. Now, I am unafraid. Even though not every day is happy and the future is uncertain, my life is precious.

I'm now happy and at peace with myself. I've made major changes and met many wonderful people. After my successful pregnancy, the Follow-Up Services Department at Craig approached me about becoming a resource person — to speak to women and men about my experiences being pregnant. It has been wonderful for me to be able to help other people with injuries and their families.

Audrey Begay

In April 2003, at my yearly re-evaluation, I enjoyed sharing my experiences as a young mother and the staff told me how proud they were of me and all that I had accomplished. At the same time, my insurance refused to cover the new wheelchair that I needed. Fortunately, because of my overall attitude as well as my need, I was chosen to receive a custom-made chair in a sponsored wheelchair giveaway program affiliated with Craig. It was a big event, and I even gave speeches — with Adrian and little Hannah by my side.

Audrey Begay lives in Lakewood, Colorado. She is a full-time mom writing her autobiography.

Life Need Not Be Easy, as Long as It is Interesting

Aline Moran
C6
Age at SCI: 60
Date of SCI: July 3, 1998
Truckee, California

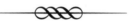

*T*he magnitude of my injury did not hit me until I got home after a three-month stay in the hospital. Although the rehab program was disorganized and left me with lots of time on my hands, my condition, C6 incomplete quadriplegia, was such that I slept much of the time.

As I began to come out of my stupor, I noticed that I was the only patient without a deputy sheriff stationed at my door. The only thing I had in common with my fellow patients was a spinal cord injury. They were young, black, single males with gang-related gunshot wounds; I was an old, white, married female. Their greatest concern, after taking care of the guy who shot them, was if and how they were going to have sex again. Post-injury sex was not high on my priority list. I had been married forty years and figured I could deal with that later.

I became very fond of my gang friends. They were just as bewildered and frightened as I. We met at the gym and gave each other encouragement. In the afternoons, we went out on the smoking porch (I don't smoke, but it was our only outdoors). Several guys, butt-side up on gurneys, had paid no attention to warnings to shift their weight regularly and had landed back in the hospital with sores. This sure motivated me to shift my weight around.

When we said goodbye, I returned to a life, difficult as it might be, without the loneliness and financial worries that would face many of these young men. As I departed, a nurse leaned over and whispered, "You're going to make it." I thought to myself, "Of course I'm going to make it." Little did I know what lay between that day and "making it."

You don't have to be paralyzed to become depressed, but it sure helps. Within a few days of returning home, depression set in.

Describing depression is like trying to describe the genius of Mozart without ever hearing his music. Your brain becomes disconnected. It is impossible to focus, concentrate, plan, or anticipate. I felt like a tethered dog that had been fed and then forgotten, and my family didn't know what to do with me. I could hear the rest of the family laughing as I lay helpless in bed staring at the ceiling.

Initially, I wasn't able to transfer in and out of bed. My only choices were to sit in an ill-fitting wheelchair that I often fell out of, or go to bed. My physical therapist offered little encouragement and knew little about the fitting of wheelchairs.

The choices in my life were by appointment only. To reach for something required calling someone. Intermittent catheterization was a huge ordeal. Bowel accidents were seismic. It was not long before resentment set in, both on my part and my family's. Self-pity and isolation quickly followed. Even if I could articulate my needs and desires, it would have been difficult for my family to respond. I wanted to be independent and productive again, but I had no idea how to accomplish that.

Then things got really bad. Depression turned to despair. Everything that identified me as a person was gone. Before my accident, I had nice looking ankles and a reasonably flat tummy. Now, my ankles looked like footballs, and, slouched down in my wheelchair, I looked pregnant. I lost all sense of proportion. The appearance of my ankles and stomach were as catastrophic to me as my ongoing respiratory insufficiency caused by broken ribs punching holes in my lungs.

I was forsaken, abandoned, a colossal burden. I craved sleep. If only

I could sleep forever. A close friend of mine, who had a similar accident, had been unable to cope and killed herself. How much worse could this get? Would this black hell ever end? If I couldn't get a handle on this, I would either die or end up in a nursing home.

The final insult was an incompetent caregiver my family had hired. Having no knowledge about caring for a quadriplegic, they had been desperate and took the first person that came along. I knew immediately that she was a disaster. In spite of her sweet disposition, she lacked the intelligence and imagination to care for me. On errands, she repeatedly got lost. When we tried grocery shopping together, I discovered that she couldn't read.

When I made the transition to an intelligent, resourceful, and experienced caregiver, my life began to change. No longer did I have to direct every move. She anticipated my needs and more. I began to eat regularly. Sadly, this came at a great price. After two almost perfect years, she was caught embezzling money from me. She is now in prison.

Nevertheless, with the daily chores of bathing, cooking, meal planning, and laundry being efficiently taken care of, I was finally able to turn my attention, however briefly, to matters so long abandoned. Not that I cared much about anything, but, just to relieve the monotony, I tried to get back to the computer. I figured that I needed to do something proactive.

Suddenly, I found that I did not have to go to sleep in the middle of the morning. This was a huge step upward. Because of an ill-fitting wheelchair, it was very uncomfortable to hold my hands on the keyboard for much more than twenty minutes at a time. Almost imperceptibly, I began to care about not caring. I became agitated and uncomfortable with my isolation and disinterest in life.

With a properly fitting wheelchair, I was able to extend my computer sessions to an hour at a time, and I began to write letters to my imaginary therapist. Each day, I would unload on him. Everything that had gone wrong the day before, however petty, got put down in words. An hour passed in a flash. I had a lot to say.

This process proved very helpful. It put things in perspective. When I read back my words, it was easy to pick the serious problems from the trivia. Indeed, there were still serious bouts of depression. I remember days when I couldn't go for more than five minutes without the reality of my condition hitting me in the face. Gradually, I could go for about a half an hour before a reality check occurred. That turned into every four hours. Now, it happens about once a day.

When I got my proper wheelchair, I also found an exercise bike that enabled me to get out on the road and ride. Prior to my injury, I got going by riding a bike first thing in the morning. Now, I was able to reintroduce an activity that had meant so much. Later, I saw a bike engineered for racing and long distance riding that would do more than any antidepressant drug to lift my spirits. I ride my Freedom Ryder almost daily.

Many of the experiences of my sixty years served me well as I began to come out of the darkness. Eight years in public office with its campaigning, lost elections, and negative news stories had taught me an important lesson in enduring humiliation.

I also forced myself to participate in some disabled sports programs. It was uncomfortable and humiliating. I asked to join a horseback-riding program geared for autistic children. I was led around like a child, but it taught me some balance both physically and emotionally.

Skiing in a bucket was initially uncomfortable and humiliating. It took an enormous effort by my family to get me on the slopes for a ski program geared toward children with physical and emotional disabilities. I was tethered and had to confine my routine to that of a child. Working with me probably provided some relief to my patient instructors.

Together with a friend, a high school swim coach, we tried various techniques until I mastered a dog-paddle crawl stroke that has enabled me to swim several laps. It was very tedious to suit up and get in the cold water, but it paid off. As with my pre-injury sports achievements, persistence led to endurance and that led to success.

Although no wallet in the world is fat enough to protect one from despair and depression, financial security helped me. Adapting my home so I could live comfortably was a major factor in coming out of my depression. Just the planning stage got my mind focused. The adaptation was long and expensive. We installed an elevator and numerous ramps, lowered sinks, and opened up a shower. My bath no longer consisted of buckets of water poured over me as I sat on a stool in the middle of a child's wading pool in the laundry room.

Using a rock climbing harness that fit around my waist and through my legs, my husband was able to pull me up onto my feet and I began "walking" a couple of hundred feet twice a day. This has had very positive results in controlling spasticity and maintaining muscle tone in my legs, and, together with a couple of hours daily in a standing frame, has eliminated any need for anti-spasticity drugs.

My decision about not using drugs was influenced by a long family history of alcohol abuse. I, myself, had misused alcohol and for the past fifteen years had not touched it. Having witnessed firsthand the agonies members of my family had endured while getting sober, I viewed any mind-altering drug as soporific and potentially addictive. Further, I felt strongly that I would need every ounce of mental acuity I could muster to deal with the challenges that faced me. My own experiences and stories of addiction and withdrawal from friends and family were enough to scare me away from antidepressant and anti-anxiety drugs. Furthermore, I was gradually coming out of the worst levels of depression.

In my third year post-injury, I began to wean myself off of caregivers by cutting down from ten hours to four. I got an adaptive van that enabled me to wheel in, transfer into the driver's seat, and drive using my hands. By installing a hands-free cell phone, I was confident enough to drive myself to town fifteen miles away, run errands, and meet friends.

Other accomplishments quickly followed. I learned to transfer to a shower bench and shower myself. I began to cook and play the piano again. I go to the gym and lift weights every other day. With a caregiver at my side, I doubt if I would have ever attempted these things.

Our family had backpacked extensively. With a special treeless saddle, I am now able to get into the backcountry on horseback. Although I used to hate the sight of horses on the trail, now I depend on horses and mules for backcountry experiences.

We used to join our university alumni group on study/travel tours. We now go independently. I miss the camaraderie but have been pleasantly surprised at the contacts we have made. Photography, fly-fishing, and birding direct our destinations. I have yet to be turned down when I contact a guide service and explain my special needs. They usually take it as a challenge and arrange innovative, interesting trips.

Some issues can never be fully resolved. My depression has evolved into periods of sadness, frustration, and self-pity that, mercifully, occur less and less frequently. My life has very little spontaneity because I can't just get up and go as I used to. Instead, I prepare a daily flight plan for myself. A forgotten detail — full gas tank, catheters, cell phone — can cause major headaches for everyone. Cameras, cooking ingredients, office supplies, phones, or clothes moved with intentions of helping me clean up, a child's bike blocking my way, or a recipe ingredient put up out of reach can cause disproportionately high levels of frustration. I constantly have to remind myself that the baking powder on the unreachable top shelf is not a big deal.

Until he retired, my husband's insurance covered the medical supplies I needed. Now that Medicare is our primary insurer, the documentation and justification demand hours, and the reimbursement procedures drive me crazy.

The anxiety associated with the prospect of a bowel or bladder accident is always present. Regulating my eating, keeping to a schedule, and listening to what few signs my body sends to my brain have reduced my accident rate to a few times a year. Using a catheter/plastic bag combination provides extraordinary flexibility.

Adjusting to a SCI has been a long, slow process of acceptance. Few people get to my age without something awful happening to them. My condition is just a little more obvious. Otherwise normal-appearing people are walking around dealing with fright, anguish, loneliness, helplessness, and panic. SCI survivors don't have a monopoly on the bad luck and capriciousness life deals us.

Aline Moran lives in Truckee, California. A graduate of Stanford University, she spent her married life in the San Joaquin Valley, where her husband practiced law and later became a judge. They have four children and ten grandchildren. Aline served two terms as a city councilwoman and vice mayor. She is a photographer, teacher (English and adult literacy), writer, and landscape designer.

Time, Time, Time:
See What's Become of Me

Bill Hiser

T10

Age at SCI: 20

Date of SCI: November 9, 1970

Lexington, Ohio

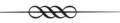

*L*ast week was a heck of a week. I was able to ...

Be a guest speaker in a 9/11 tribute for our community.

Teach Sunday school at church.

Host a full house at our bed and breakfast for a week.

Play and even win some of the ten games of ping-pong that I played with my fourteen-year-old son.

Help my fifth grade daughter master her multiplication tables and watch a beautiful ten-year-old child change in front of my eyes.

Encourage my wife as she prepares to run her first marathon.

Truly, I am a blessed man.

If you would have told me about any of the above thirty-two years ago in the intensive care ward in a military hospital in the Republic of Viet Nam, I would have asked the nurse to give you a shot of morphine. Clearly, you would have been out of your mind.

The day after my twentieth birthday, our squad walked into an ambush. I was shot with an AK-47. The bullet entered under my left armpit and stopped just short of my spinal cord at T10. As I lay on the ground, I could see blood spurt out of the wound. I had seen dead men, and I thought I was one. I was angry that I wasn't going to see my family and my girlfriend again — or drive my 1968 Mustang. But, I had become a Christian in junior high, and I was excited that if I was going to die, I would see heaven.

My world became very simple. Breathe in and out. Stay awake. Don't close my eyes.

Four days later, I woke up in great pain. The nurse told me I was in a Stryker frame. The Doctor told me I would never walk again. My brain told me my life was over. The morphine dulled the pain, but did nothing for my broken heart. I cried, I prayed, and I tried to talk God into a deal. And I listened to the boy next to me as he was dying. He cried for his mom and for some Jujubes. During those days in intensive care, I spent my deepest, darkest hours. Ever. I believe God broke me down and shaped me for what was to come.

Saigon to Japan to Walter Reed hospital in Washington, D.C. America — how good it felt to be back in America. To be back in the "World," and know I was going to live. I had a bed by the window, and I'd watch our floor nurse drive up in her Porsche. I fell in love with the idea of her, her car, and me — headed for points west. That didn't happen. More importantly, my loving family came from Ohio.

After the tears came laughter, then more tears. Home-cooked food and Jones' potato chips, school news from my sisters, Sally and Jill, and hearing how our old farmhouse was getting made ready for me. My dad and mom made many eleven-hour trips just to spend a few short hours with me. My family's love and support helped heal my spirit.

Cleveland Veterans Administration Hospital was next. Out of the Stryker frame into a bed, out of the bed into a wheelchair, off the floor, and into the sunshine. We paras mixed drinks and lit smokes for the quads. As the ashes fell off his cigarette and onto the front of his shirt, Dr. "D" told me what my sex life was going to be. As a para, the physical parts weren't going to happen. Sex and love were really in your head anyway, and I'd soon get over it. As far as kids, there was always adoption. That night I went to bed feeling empty, angry, and cheated.

June 4th became my Independence Day. Home with no weekend pass in my hand. No parade for this veteran — but a meal fit for a king from my mom, a ramp from my friend, and new bathroom from my dad. I let my hair grow and dated a beautiful hippie girl who dressed in bell-bottoms and tie-dyed tops. That fall, she moved to St. Louis, and I headed for college in Phoenix.

At Arizona State University, my self-worth started to return through using my mind and being successful in the classroom. People looked past the chair and wanted to know me, and I started to wake up to the "disability movement." It started as only it could for me — with sports. I was like any other kid that grew up in the 1960s — sports with my sisters till the yell, "Dinnersready!" When the seasons changed, the games changed but playing was constant. Sitting in a wheelchair and throwing a Frisbee wasn't enough. There had to be a "testing" of skill and of heart against other guys. Inside, I still felt like I was being measured and found wanting. With sports, I could prove I was whole.

A group of us started to shoot baskets at the intramural gym. Soon our wheelchair basketball team was born. We needed gym time. To get it, we had to take it from someone. We felt our first bit of prejudice. The able-bodied athletes had to be shown we too were athletes. We fought the prejudice by becoming a team with real skill. Our practices were a time of crashing boards and smashing bodies. Then, afterwards, there was time for talking about our lives.

How important that time of pizza, beer, and talking became. We started with just teammates but soon wives and girlfriends started coming. We would talk about everything under the sun. Over time, we became a community. We cared about, looked out for, and tried to help solve each others' problems. Soon, other students with disabilities showed up and become part of our group. Some nights very little basketball was discussed; but, we'd be the last group to leave when it was closing time.

Five years later, I graduated with a degree in education and went looking for my first junior high teaching job. I had spent time teaching Sunday school before the war and enjoyed it. I knew teaching was going to be a good fit for me. Besides, I like the fact that when a junior high student stands up, he or she is just tall enough so we can talk eye to eye.

Mesa (Arizona) Junior High, room 509, became my second home. I was single and all the love and energy I put into my students came back to me ten-fold. It was a time of magic.

Four years into teaching I got a call from our guidance counselor, Ralph Moreno. We needed to help the students with disabilities feel more accepted and to educate the other kids. Ideas started to come and soon we were ready. We put teachers in wheelchairs, had a neat assembly and wheelchair races at lunchtime for students, and "Night of the Wheel" — a wheelchair basketball game. Teachers played against the Arizona State University team. The night was a fundraiser and an awareness raiser for the kids, parents, and community. Soon, other schools in the area started to do their own "awareness events."

In 1980, I turned thirty, after ten years of using a wheelchair. Friends took me out to a cowboy bar to celebrate. As I sat and watched all the young, good-looking cowboys and cowgirls dance, I became heartsick. I had played by the rules. I had graduated and had a great job — everyone thought I was a success. But inside, I was weary to the bone of being in a wheelchair. I wanted out. I wanted to walk and run and dance. I just wanted to stand up. And if that wasn't going to happen, then I wanted to hurt someone. The code of the West broke when I put a lit cigarette out in a pitcher of beer. The cowboy hit me and I hit the floor. I waited until the bouncer got there to get up. I was escorted out, got into my car, and drove home. In the garage, behind the wheel, I sat and cried.

That night was a crossroads for me. It hit me that after ten years in a chair I wasn't going to get up and walk. This was my life. My body wasn't going to get better. From now until I died, I was going to be that guy in the chair. But then, the next thoughts changed me. It was the way it was. It was okay. It sure wasn't my first choice, but it was okay. I was okay. But my friends and I had been living like God wasn't important. I knew that was wrong. Without God, all that had happened to me would just be random chance, and I just couldn't believe that. I knew I had to get back to a church and get back to God. It was past time.

In 1984, I met the woman who would become my wife. Ellen worked in a hotel in Cape May, New Jersey, where I had taken a summer job. On the way home from our first date, I got lost and pulled over to figure how to get home. Ellen thought I was going to try something less than honorable. Hand on the door handle, she knew she could outrun me if I did try something. All summer long, I did try something — and our love blossomed. In the fall, Ellen flew out to visit my life in Mesa. My friends loved her — and amazingly, she said yes. On June 22, 1985, we were married. I became husband of a beautiful, tall, blonde, and very talented woman. She quickly turned my Mesa house into our home, and just as quickly became the love of my life and my best friend.

In 1987, after ten years of teaching, we were ready for a new chapter in our lives. We moved back to Ohio. We bought a farm and turned a one-hundred-and-ten-year-old house into a cozy bed and breakfast. It is hard work, and many of our guests have become great friends. Zac was born in 1988. Watching Ellen's body change month by month and the long hours of her pushing and squeezing my hand were very special. I had become a family man. Holding him in my arms, I was amazed by the love I felt for him and overwhelmed with the memories of all that had come before. Hannah was born in 1992 and our beautiful redhead has, just this year, outgrown my lap. They both can pop wheelies in my spare chair. Along with Ellen we play, fight, and love just like any other family. I wish Dr. "D" were alive to see how wrong he was.

In 1995, I started working for the Independent Living Center of North Central Ohio. I felt it was time to pay back for all the good things that had happened to me. Meeting real people with real disabilities brought me back to the disability community in a big way. I had been a man with a disability living in an able-bodied world. Now, my list of friends grew to people who worked in sheltered workshops and tried to live on $490 a month. Our great staff fights for small victories and dreams big dreams. I've wheeled up new ramps that allow people to get out of their homes and helped provide hearing aids, wheelchairs — and hope. School assemblies, wheelchair bowling, and playing Santa Claus at the Christmas party are all parts of my life — and none of the kids notices that Santa uses a chair. The family is included in everything we do. Each day, something new and exciting comes into our office.

Thirty-two years of using a wheelchair — the greatest gift is time. Time to heal. Time to grow. Time to attempt, to fail, to succeed. Time to find your life and, most importantly, to live it. Time to find God's will. Time to make a difference.

I am not the same man as that twenty-year-old boy who was so sure his life was over so many years ago. In my life, there was change and change and more change. Today, I continue to lead a good, full life.

To God be the glory, great things He has done.

Bill Hiser lives on a farm outside of Lexington, Ohio with his wife, Ellen, and their two children, Zac and Hannah. His days are filled doing many different things, and he enjoys spending some of his down time with his dog Rocko and cat Fred.

Living Well Is the Best Revenge

Gordon Palmer
C4-5
Age at SCI: 18
Date of SCI: May 29, 1977
Tallahassee, Florida

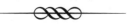

Twenty-six years ago, I never thought I'd still be using this wheelchair in 2003. After my accident on May 29, 1977, my future was very uncertain. Although my functional abilities and sensation haven't changed much, my life sure has. Even though I still have no feeling from the chest down and from just above my elbows and have very limited use of my arms and wear splints on both hands/wrists, my life is pretty good. I'm an attorney for a state agency, own a modified home and van, have friends, travel, and am involved in the community.

I was injured in a single car accident two weeks before my high school graduation. I passed out while driving home after a rock concert and drinking too much. The last thing I remember is getting on the interstate highway at 4 a.m. The next thing I remember is waking up in a hospital a week later with a C4-5 injury. I was told that the car went into the highway median, flipped over, and threw me and my friend out and onto the median. I was also told that I was alert and talking after the accident, but I sure don't remember it. Fortunately, my friend had only minor injuries.

When I woke up in the hospital bed, I couldn't move anything. I had no feeling in most of my body and my long hair had been completely shaved off. My first thought was "Man, I *really* fucked up this time!" I was very worried about what was going to happen to me and whether I would get better. I didn't receive one of those speeches about how I would never walk again. Information regarding my condition seemed to be minimal, as if the doctors were afraid to say anything to me.

I didn't know anybody with a disability and never even thought about something like this happening. I had a very active life — surfing, water ski-ing, boating, skateboarding, and partying. My accident was a huge shock.

For a long time, my emotional state was one of bewilderment or cluelessness. Being on a respirator for the first six weeks and not being able to talk didn't help. But even after I got off of it and went through six months of rehab, I felt like I was in a new and completely different world.

When I moved from intensive care to a spinal cord injury rehabilita-tion facility, I learned a lot from therapists, especially the importance of range of motion exercises and skin care. I also learned by talking with other patients. Although I did not realize it at the time, it was an informal peer support system. It was very helpful to discuss problems and concerns with people who were going through the same things and trying to figure out what to do. And, I made some good friends who I am still in touch with.

Fortunately, I had a lot of family support. My parents, my sister, and two brothers visited me almost every day and demonstrated their love in many ways. Once I was home, for the first five or six years, my dad got me up for my morning routine before he went to work and put me in bed most nights. My family members took me to therapy and college classes, and were there whenever I needed something.

I also had a lot of support from my friends. My friends came to visit me regularly in the hospital and after I got home. Several friends organized a big benefit barbecue with local bands. With the proceeds from this and a benefit my church had for me, my family was able to purchase a van with a lift, making it much easier for me to get around.

Despite all this support, there were many times when I wished I had died. The change was so sudden and so severe — to go from running around and being almost completely independent to being almost totally dependent was frustrating and depressing. My bladder and bowel problems only compounded these feelings. Sometimes, I thought about ending it all. Since we lived on a lake, the method was in my back yard. But I decided I had already put my parents, family, and friends through too much. I also believed that things would get better — probably because I am an optimist and did not have my whole life planned out. I just kept going and hoped that tomorrow would be a better day.

Getting used to and accepting my disability took years. I believe that it was easier to accept my disability because I was driving and the accident was my fault; I had no one else to blame.

After high school, I had planned to go to the Netherlands as an exchange student for a year. Then I was going to work and surf for a year or two while figuring out what to do with my life. Since the trip and surfing were out, I went to a local community college and then to a university that was twenty-three miles from my family home. Although transportation was sometimes a problem, I managed to work things out with friends, old and new. So many people were driving my van that my insurance company would have dropped me if they ever found out. Disabled Student Services provided note takers and other assistance; the state vocational rehabilitation agency paid my tuition and gave me a book allowance.

College was a good place to get adjusted. I was busy doing something productive. And, there were plenty of attractive women there and a lot of breaks. In my junior year, I started thinking about law school because I didn't think I was ready for the real work world and realized I would need a higher income for all of my disability-related expenses.

Law school was tough because it involved a completely different teaching and testing style. Many times, my fear of failure motivated me. Sometimes, I felt that I was in over my head — but I persevered. I often used the saying "you have only failed when you have failed to try" to motivate myself — I still use it regularly.

Law school meant a new city and living independently. I had doubts about whether I could do it; but, I knew it would be the best thing for me. I lived in a center for independent living residential program that provided accessible subsidized housing, utilities, and transportation. Once again, other people with spinal cord injuries were my support system. We shared many problems as well as personal care assistants — and more than a few beers — during the years I lived there.

Except for summers in high school, I had never worked full time. Fortunately, my supportive employer appreciated that I wanted the job and was trying my best. My employer installed an electric door opener, and I obtained a workstation from Vocational Rehabilitation. I worked hard and the continued support and encouragement of my family and friends helped keep me going.

I don't think I've ever adjusted to my bladder and bowel problems. I learned to tolerate, correct, and minimize them — and keep on going. Knowledge of the alternatives to not working has kept me going. I did not want to live with my parents for the rest of their lives or end up in a nursing home or some government-subsidized housing program dependent on Social Security. I wanted opportunities to go places, do things, and be respected.

It is really true that knowledge is power. And, it doesn't have to be knowledge from a university or law school. Other people with disabilities continue to be one of my best sources of knowledge. I've learned about procedures, products, and what is accessible. I also get information by reading and using the Internet.

Disability specific issues like accessibility or personal care are a lot to contend with. Add in the ordinary problems of life, and it can be almost overwhelming. I focus on the positive — that my injury was not worse than it was and that I'm still alive. I also try to learn from my mistakes and from others. I put the past behind me and keep going.

Thousands of times my mind has been flooded with "if only" thoughts. But, I realize history cannot be changed and it does no good to dwell on the past. I'm stuck with my injury, and I try to make the best of it by getting out and making life worth living. I enjoy being with my family and friends, my girlfriend (when I have one), traveling, going to nightclubs, community events, surfing the Internet, e-mail, music, movies, going to college football games, and hanging out at the beach or pool on warm sunny days.

There have been a number of rough times. Dealing with my urological problems have been some of the roughest. I spent the first eleven years dealing with external/condom catheters that made my life hell sometimes because, as a quad, I couldn't take care of the problems (leaks) myself. The next twelve years were better because I used a super-pubic catheter. Then I had more problems and had to get an illio-conduit. The first year with it was hell and the worst year medically in twenty years. However, after surgery to get rid of scar tissue that resulted from the original illio-conduit surgery, it's been great. I also have had to deal with a spinal cord cyst and surgery three years after my accident, and then losing my mom to cancer a year later.

Besides occasional problems with personal care assistants, health, and finances, women and sexuality have been big issues for me. Before my accident, I was a stud. Thinking with my "little head" instead of my big one was also a contributing factor in my accident. I felt so inadequate sexually after my accident. It didn't help that I was using an external catheter. But, with time and a willing and understanding partner, I learned different procedures and adjusted. Finding willing partners can be challenging — but they are out there. Fortunately, there is now more information about options as well as discussions of sexuality than when I was first injured. Patience, perseverance, a sense of humor, adaptability, and the willingness to try different methods have all helped.

I have found that it helps to be assertive. I've also developed a toughness that I will survive and prosper despite all the disability-related bullshit. I've learned to let the small stuff go. I take care of myself and focus on what I need to do to get where I want to be. Over time, I have developed a positive attitude and have realized that life can be good.

I'm glad I'm alive. Living well really is the best revenge, and it doesn't necessarily require a lot of money. For me, it's a lot about being healthy, having options to do what I want, and simplifying things to minimize prob-lems. As an attorney with a state agency, I usually only work forty hours each week, get four weeks annual leave and three weeks sick leave, and have comprehensive medical insurance. To simplify life, I live near my office. Besides less traffic and commuting time, if necessary, I can drive my wheel-chair home or to work. Having a live-in personal care assistant, I'm not con-stantly scheduling people and have more flexibility. All these factors help me have the freedom to do what I want.

The Americans with Disabilities Act has helped me by making places more accessible with curb cuts, ramps, and accessible parking. I remember the nuisance of being lifted up curbs and steps and taking two parking spots so the van lift could be lowered. In college, I was called "the road warrior" because I spent so much time driving my wheelchair in the road because there were no curb cuts.

Advances in technology have also made my life easier. My current wheelchair is more durable and reliable, can recline or tilt, and has a quiet motor, an electric leg bag emptier, and tire inserts to prevent flat tires. Voice dictation computer software, advances in van modifications, and remote con-trols help too. And, with the growth in the adaptive equipment field, I have several manufacturers to choose from for most of the products that I need.

Public awareness has also made my life easier because people have more accepting attitudes. When I was first injured, the public didn't know about spinal cord injuries and had no clue why I needed a wheelchair. And, hardly anyone discussed spinal cord injury cure research.

Most of all, I remember that it's the journey, not the destination, that counts. Although the journey can be difficult, the trip is worthwhile and can be enjoyable.

Gordon Palmer lives in Tallahassee, Florida. He is a full-time attorney with a state agency and volunteers with several disability-related organizations. He is single, a weekend hedonist, and a big Florida State Seminoles football fan.

Ups, Downs, and Breakthroughs

Kirk Feyerabend
T5-6
Age at SCI: 44
Date of SCI: June 18, 2000
Pleasanton, California

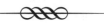

A s a forty-four-year-old, divorced, childless, and somewhat lonely man, I had decided the year 2000 was going to be different. I was healthy, attractive, making good money, and lived in a great town with wonderful neighbors and lots of friends. But something was missing. I wanted a partner, a lover, and soul mate. On New Year's Eve 1999, I was convinced things were going to change for the better. In the wee hours of the new millennium, it started. An affair with a stunningly beautiful tall, blonde, blue-eyed woman began that night! The fact that she was still legally married with two children bothered me — but not enough to stop seeing her.

The economy was booming, and I loved my job. Motorcycling, my passion since childhood, was dominating my free time. I commuted to work, rain or shine, on a motorcycle and raced on tracks and off road on the weekends. By May, things were really looking up. I had plans for the coming summer — races, camping, riding, and play — with most including my new girlfriend and her kids.

One weekend in June, in an instant, I went from euphoric optimism to absolute despair. I was riding my dirt bike when I came upon a huge tree stump whose roots created a nasty jump in the trail. I was going way too fast and flew over the handlebars — hitting my head on a rock as my back smashed into a log with an audible "crunch." Even before I stopped flopping down the trail, I knew I was hurt bad. I came to rest on my stomach in the middle of the cold, wet trail with a horrifying sensation. I could not feel anything from the chest down.

Four hours later, I was finally strapped to a gurney in a Coast Guard helicopter in a state of shock. My body temperature was dangerously low from lying on the cold ground for so long waiting for help. X-rays confirmed the worst: thoracic vertebra 5 was pulverized; T4, 6, 7 and 8 were fractured. After I was stabilized, I was flown to Santa Clara Valley Medical Center to await surgery and to start rehab.

"Paralysis!" "Paraplegic!" The words screamed inside my head. I knew little about spinal cord injury. I was getting an education, like it or not. After surgery, I was eager to start rehab. Yet, in the back of my mind, I was hopeful I would regain full function. The doctors told me I was a T5-6 complete and that the chances for recovery were not impossible but highly unlikely. "Brain and spinal cord cells do not regenerate and there is no cure, so get used to the new you" was the message I heard — but did not want to accept.

I felt my situation was unfair to my girlfriend. Since she was getting a divorce, to expect her to stick by my side just didn't feel right. To protect my ego, I took the initiative. I gathered up the strength and through tears told her, "It is okay to walk away. This is not your battle." She soon stopped visiting.

I was never religious. I always admired people with strong religious convictions. I wanted to believe — but it is not something you can fake. I tried anyway. In my darkest moments, I would pray to God to come and take me, to end my misery. "Please God, let me die." He wasn't listening. Okay, fine, I can take care of this on my own. I'll go through the motions in rehab, get out, go home to where I have a couple handguns, and kill myself. At times, I was shocked by my simple plan. I never had a suicidal thought before the accident. Now, I had a plan with the means?

Thanks to my family, friends, doctors, nurses, and therapists, my plan faded. I began to realize they were investing tremendous amounts of time, energy, and patience in my rehabilitation — so that I could live an independent, productive life. To waste all that with a gun shot to the head would be letting so many people down.

A couple of weeks post-rehab, friends invited me to a motorcycle race in San Diego. My home was undergoing remodeling, and I was sleeping in the living room, taking sponge baths, and doing my bowel program in a bucket. A real shower or bath in a hotel room sounded good, and seeing my racing buddies would be great. So, I was going on my first out of town trip, solo. My spirits were high.

I made flight arrangements and called to arrange hotel accommodations with wheelchair access. Since they didn't have roll-in showers, I asked if they had a transfer bench for the tub. They replied, "Yeah, uh, we have one of those." I was set for my first flight and first hotel stay.

My friends met me at the airport, and we went to check in. Surprise! There was no transfer bench — and it was Friday night with no way to get one! I had learned how to get in a tub with a bench in rehab but had no idea what to do without one. I told my friend, Carl, I might need help in the morning getting in and out of the tub. A minor setback, but we were off to meet more friends for dinner. I was still on a high.

Early Saturday morning, I woke up to change positions and noticed a nasty smell. I pulled back the covers to find I had had diarrhea during in the night! I couldn't believe it. My first bout of diarrhea happens in a strange hotel room. I was pissed. Cursing and wondering what was I going to do, I transferred onto my wheelchair, messing up the cushion cover. I called Carl, waking him. "Carl, there has been a slight change of plans. Helping me into the tub is going to be much more unpleasant than you expected." I was literally covered in crap.

Carl tried to console me saying, "This is nothing; I have two boys." I said, "That's family stink — not friend stink. There is a big difference." He laughed, helped me into the tub, and left. I started the clean-up process — fill the tub, drain the tub, fill the tub, drain tub, and so on. After getting myself and my chair cleaned-up, I realized I had no way to summon Carl. I was sitting in the tub feeling about as low as possible.

I began thinking, "If I can just get my butt up on the ledge of the tub." That didn't work. "Let's try putting my feet out first and — ta da, I'm almost there! Next, I had to transfer from the ledge to the chair. I removed the cushion so it was not as large a step. Grunt, and I was there. My first tub-to-chair transfer on my own! Getting out of a tub is much harder than getting in.

After a great day at the races, I was feeling good again. My brother joined us, and I was peaking on my emotional roller coaster! But then, I woke up Sunday morning to the same mess! Now I was really pissed! How can this happen two nights in a row? The shame, frustration, and anger were in full swing. However, it was not quite as big a mess, and I knew how to handle it on my own. I got cleaned-up in time to make curtain call, and we were off to the track. Seeing all my friends and being at the races where I love to be was just a great experience. I was emotionally on top again.

Monday morning, same thing! Now I was beyond pissed. I was thinking if there is a God, why would He do this to anyone? My cursing was pretty intense. I'm sure my neighbors in the hotel must have heard me. This routine was getting really old. But, at the same time it, was getting easier to deal with.

I was cleaned up and ready to go to the airport on time. At check out, my friend's wife, Kim, insisted on talking with the manager about the lack of a transfer bench. He gave up nothing, staring back at her with arms crossed and jaw locked. When she finished and stomped out to the car, the manager turned to me and said, "I've already been in touch with our attorneys and our hotel meets all the requirements of the ADA." He continued, "I understand you had some 'accidents' and we will have to replace the mattress and linens. You will be billed for these items." I was stunned. After a while, I was able to mumble, "I suppose that is only fair," and I rolled out of there.

Since this happened about the time Clint Eastwood was being sued by a woman in a wheelchair for access to something or other, I sensed there was a bit of a backlash against the disability community. I bet that SOB hotel manager was thinking I was posturing for a lawsuit. That really got me down because I'm one who thinks we are a litigation-crazed society, looking for somebody else to pay for our self-inflicted misery.

Before my flight, I had plenty of time to reflect on what had happened. I had experienced intense humiliation, shame, frustration, and anger. I also experienced tenderness and understanding — but those feelings were being run over by the negative emotions. I swore I would never leave town again. I was feeling pretty miserable, fighting back tears, when a remarkable thing happened.

As I sat waiting for my flight, a strange-looking, three-wheeled wheelchair came past with a quad pushing it from his own chair. I recognized the light-weight three-wheeler as a racing chair. Then another one came into the waiting lounge, then another one! Next, in walked a beautiful young woman wearing shorts — a double amputee proudly showing off her artificial lower legs! Pretty soon the room was full of people with various disabilities.

Wondering what was going on, I stopped the first guy to ask. As he gave me a bone-crushing handshake, he introduced himself as Burt Burns. I was impressed because I saw that he is a low-level quad. He told me this group had been training in San Diego and was on the way to the Los Angeles airport to catch a non-stop flight to Sydney, Australia, to compete in the 2000 Para-lympics! I was completely blown away!

I started peppering Burt with questions, "LA to Sydney is one of the longest non-stop flights there is. How do you go to the bathroom? How do you get around in the plane? What about the jet lag?" He was polite and answered as best he could. But, his interest had shifted to a very attractive blonde in a short skirt with a very European look. He rolled over to her and chatted her up. She and her friends were German tourists checking out the Western United States. There I was sitting in the airport talking with a group of Paralympic athletes and some German tourists. We talked about what they thought of the U. S., about disabilities in general, and how people with disabilities are viewed in Germany.

After meeting a guy with an injury worse than mine who was going to compete in the Paralympics and was still able to flirt with pretty girls, I began to think that my difficulties of the past couple of days were not all that bad. In fact, the whole emotional roller coaster taught me that I was allowing myself to be dragged up and down emotionally by events happening around me.

I used to get bummed out when I would see my ex-girl friend with her new guy. I mean, why not? Now, I'm a divorced, childless, somewhat lonely, paraplegic man. However, I prefer to think of myself as a bright, competent, capable, and desirable man.

By the way, I never did get a bill for the mattress.

Kirk Feyerabend lives and plays in Pleasonton, California. He works in the Silicon Valley in sales and marketing, and is a mentor in Santa Clara Valley Medical Center's mentor program. He continues his involvement in motor sports with a motorcycle customized with retractable outriggers and races a 125 kart with hand controls.

Holding Together: A Newborn Life

Samantha Kimball-Fell
C6-7
Age at SCI: 24
Date of SCI: October 12, 1993
Austin, Texas

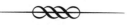

*A*t twenty-four, I had it all figured out — I was newly married, with a three-year plan. I would work in Austin until Thanksgiving, not announcing my plans to leave until I received the promotion I knew I would soon get. This would show my new employer that I was a hot young engineering talent with management potential. Then, I would join my husband in Alabama where he worked as a golf course superintendent, get a job at the local Sony plant, play a lot of free golf, work for a few years, and then start having babies when I turned twenty-seven. That way I could have two before I was thirty. That was my plan.

It all changed on the morning of October 12, 1993. Driving to work down a back country road, something jumped in front of my car. It was most likely a raccoon, but it could have been an armadillo. It was still dark so I am not sure. Whatever it was startled me enough that I swerved to avoid it. I ran my car off the road and flipped it onto its roof. The impact of my head hitting the ceiling shattered my C7 vertebra and caused C6 to shift. By the time EMS got to me, my vital signs were pretty low. I found out later that I could have died if someone equipped with a cell phone had not been following behind me.

I remember being in the ambulance and the emergency room, but I don't remember being able to give them the phone numbers of my sister and my parents or explain that my husband was out of state. They took me straight from the ER to surgery to fuse my vertebrae. My husband flew in from Alabama, my parents drove up from San Antonio, and my in-laws drove down from Dallas. I spent eight days in the intensive care unit, mostly sleeping.

I was in a regular hospital room by the time I started to grasp what had happened. I could not turn my head or move anything but my arms, and they were so weak that I couldn't even lift them up to wipe my nose. With all the nursing activity and noise, I couldn't sleep. I was desperate to take a shower; I still had blood in my hair from the accident.

There was a lot of business to conduct once I regained my senses. There was arranging my leave of absence from work and my short-term disability benefits, arranging where I would go for rehab, and getting a power of attorney so my husband and mother could conduct my affairs. I could not hold a tissue much less a pen to sign the power of attorney, so they put the pen in my mouth and I made an "X" on the line with tears in my eyes.

This was not supposed to be happening to me. What did I ever do to deserve this? This was supposed to be one of the happiest times in my life. Bill and I had been waiting to get married, and we were ready to enjoy our life together. Instead I was lying in a hospital bed, unable to move while I thought of all the newlywed sex we were not going to have and my future children that were never going to exist. What would my life be now? To add insult to injury, I did not get my promotion because of my medical leave. I was screwed.

The next week, I was transferred to the rehab hospital. I was glad to be there. It was a lot nicer, and the food was better. They kept me busy from eight to five every day. I worked my ass off. Even "recreational" therapy usually involved lifting weights or pushing around the grounds in my wheelchair. When they weren't running me ragged with physical activity, I was being educated about my disability and realized that I had really done a number on myself. I learned about all the other bodily functions I had destroyed in addition to my ability to walk. One day they showed us a film with people talking about their lives after disability. They were saying that their life was just as good as before, they had grown as a person, there were still 9,000 out of 10,000 things they could do, etc. I thought they were full of shit.

I didn't mind all the activity because when I was busy I did not have time to think. It was the time I spent alone in my room that was the most difficult part of rehab. That's when I thought about how pathetic I was. I could not do anything for myself. I had ruined my life. I cried every day.

I was released from rehab on Christmas Eve, the end of the sixty days of inpatient rehab that my insurance would cover. It was also the general consensus among my therapists that they had done as much as they could for me. Leaving the hospital was difficult. I always thought that when people leave the hospital it is because they were cured. I was far from cured.

Bill was still working in Alabama since we needed his insurance to pay for outpatient therapy, so I went to live with my parents in San Antonio. This is where my adjustment process really began. I was twenty-four and totally dependent on my parents to feed me, bathe me, dress me, and put me to bed. I had no idea what the future would hold for me. It seemed like I could not do anything for myself, and I was very frustrated. I had to learn to have a lot of patience, either waiting for someone to help me or else struggling through tasks on my own. Trying to accomplish things on my own turned out to be important. I realized I could do some things I didn't think I could do — like holding a pen without an assistive device, picking items up off the floor and putting my bra on without help. I began to be able to do more and more for myself.

About a month later, I moved back to Austin. My sister and I moved into an accessible house she had found. I had someone come help me in the mornings, I went to therapy during the day, and my sister helped me in the evenings after work. I would get home before she did, so I had several hours alone each day, during which I was forced to fend for myself.

One day I made some microwave popcorn. It took me about thirty minutes to get it out, open it, and put it in the microwave, but I was proud of myself. This was a major victory. If no one was there to cook for me, I now knew I would not starve.

I went back to work part time six months after the accident. That summer Bill moved back from Alabama, and my sister moved out.

The next few years were full of little victories as I found I could do more and more. It just took me three times longer than most people. Those years were also filled with a lot of failures, frustration, and feelings of inadequacy. From the time my husband moved back from Alabama, he had become my primary caretaker, which was difficult for both of us. It was hard for him to watch me struggle. He gave up his career to take care of me, the house, and our personal affairs, enabling me to work full time while he stayed home. Other people saw him as "not working." I was frustrated and angry a lot. I wanted a husband, not a nurse, and I would get mad at him for things like the house not being kept to my satisfaction.

I believe he was depressed for a long time after my accident. He did not get the support he needed because people were more concerned about me. Whenever he tried to talk to people about how he was feeling all he got was "Well, how do you think she feels?" or, "Why don't you just leave her?" I had no support to offer him; I had my own problems. I found myself thinking terrible things about the man I supposedly loved and did not feel good about it. We both drank a lot and fought viciously on several occasions. We were headed for divorce.

It is hard to say why we did not split up. I think a lot of it was pure stubbornness. Even though we had only been married for six weeks prior to my accident, we had been together for six years before that. Neither one of us was willing to easily give up on a relationship in which we had invested so much. He took his marriage vow of "in sickness and in health" very seriously.

We decided to see a marriage counselor. His office was on the second floor of a building with no elevator, so my husband carried me up the stairs. As he carried me back down the stairs after the session, he tripped near the bottom. I hit my head pretty hard, and he damn near broke his leg. It was a good thing he didn't because we would have laid there on the sidewalk until someone came along. I think we both realized at that point that we could not rely on others to help. We decided to forget the counselor; we would work it out on our own.

I stopped expecting him to be perfect and realized I would be lost without him. When we fought and he got to the edge of leaving, I would ask him to please stay, and we would talk things out. Once he worked through his depression, he was able to see that, underneath the frustration, I was still the same girl he married. We quit blaming my injury for everything that was not working.

Bill and I are still married and have a newborn son.

I can remember the day, seven years after my injury, that I finally realized I was "over it." I had volunteered to give a guest lecture to an engineering class at my alma mater. I loaded my laptop into the car and drove the two hours to College Station. When I got there, I unloaded my laptop, gave the lecture and had lunch at my favorite place, all without incident. It was a nice Spring day so I decided to take my time on the way back. I enjoyed the drive, stopping to read the historical markers along the road that I had always whizzed by before. I was almost home when I got to thinking that I was pretty pleased with myself for making the trip alone. I then realized that I was doing the same things that I would have been doing had I never been injured and that I wasn't angry about being in a chair anymore. I thought about my life as a line. My accident knocked me off that line. But as the years went by, I was slowly working my way back to the line. I will never get on the same line, but I realized that I could be on one that was just as good.

There are now things I want in my life more than to walk again. That is how I know I have adjusted. I wish to never get divorced, to have a career where the work I do can make a difference in someone's life, and for the health of my family, friends, and pets.

The main thing I wanted in my life was a child. We had been trying to have a baby for some time. Last year we had a son that was stillborn four months premature — at which point the day I was injured became the second worst day of my life, but that's a whole other story. Then on September 19, my son, Matthew, arrived in this world safe and sound. A wish come true.

For many years, every birthday, every first-star-at-night, every coin in a fountain, every wishbone break, the wish was always the same: "Dear God, please let me have my body back and be whole again." I don't make that wish anymore.

Samantha Kimball-Fell lives in Austin, Texas with her husband, son, and two dogs. She recently earned her MBA and is embarking on a new career in healthcare management. She enjoys reading, quilting, spending time outdoors, and watching football. Samantha once watched fifteen college football games in one day. (It was great!)

Take the Pain

Mark Mathew Braunstein
L2-3
Age at SCI: 39
Date of SCI: August 6, 1990
Quaker Hill, Connecticut

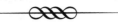

On my thirty-ninth birthday, sober but celebratory, I dived off a footbridge into a river and emerged awaiting a wheelchair. I shattered my T12 vertebra and injured that fragile bundle of nerves called the spinal cord. Diagnosis: paralysis. Not everywhere, just below the waist. Prognosis: paralysis. Not forever, just the rest of my life.

Though I seldom leave things unfinished or undone, it was my good fortune that my spinal cord injury was incomplete, that my cord was not severed, and that during rehab, my functional level progressed to L2 and L3 (and later to L4 and L5). During rehab, I began to take a stand against SCI. And one year post-injury, I began to ambulate with crutches and leg braces. I still wheel at home and at my workplace, and do nearly everything I used to do, just lower. But I continue to crutch everywhere else in between, and go nearly everywhere I used to go, just slower.

My mind dwells inside my body, but my life dwells more inside my mind. My body matters, but my mind matters more. Although my body is broken, my mind is not broken, and so my life is not broken.

When tragedy strikes, the stricken can choose to live with it, or to die from it, or to cry over it, or to laugh at it. I choose to laugh. Sure, early on, I suffered some sorrow and much pain. And sure, on some days, I contemplated suicide over my loss of a whole body that abruptly had been halved. But on other days, I did the math and added up that half a body is more than none. Indecisive, I made a secret pact with myself, the one person I could trust to keep a secret. I placed myself on a two-year waitlist. If then not fully recovered, I would reconsider suicide. Two years later, I only half-recovered my lower body, yet fully resumed my life. I half-forgot my past, and fully forgot my pact.

Now, more than thirteen years post-injury, my every step contributes to a journey from there to here, from can't to can, from injury to rehab, from disability to recovery. My journey includes some hyperbolic detours and humiliating downturns, especially because paraplegia is not just about "walk." It impacts four other four-letter words, namely "feel" plus the three sacral functions. Initially, all four took a hike.

Pardon my bedpan humor, but I still "pray for piss." I don't feel my penis, yet I do feel my fingers and do feel my tongue. So, I prefer to make love to a woman the way a woman makes love to a woman. "Come" never did come back, but ejaculation and orgasm are anti-climatic compared to being tireless in bed. Some call it tantric yoga. I call it paraplegia.

Now about "number two." Until my body hotwired its toilet training, accidents often reduced me to a whimpering fool. Other adults have accidents too, but they don't have to sit in them. During my third year post-injury, I slowly got my shit together — literally. I regained bowel function by sheer luck of the draw, but also by perseverance, having remained steadfast in my renunciation of suppositories, they being pharmaceutical drugs. Had I used and thereby become dependent upon them, my bowel function might have verged on the edge of recovery, but I never would have known it.

Prior to my injury, I had abstained from pharmaceutical drugs for seventeen years. After SCI, I avoid them still. Even the painkillers. Especially the painkillers. I abstained from them even during the calamitous first week while immobilized in a Stryker frame, that human rotisserie in which its occupant is flipped every two hours. Each flip inflicted excruciating pain, but I endured the pain.

But why endure the pain? Because most analgesics kill all sensations, both painful and pleasurable. Because drugs that inhibit feelings of sensation, inhibit feelings of emotion too. One way to hasten healing is to feel love — your own love of self, and others' love of you. Others who? Others tending to and taking care of you — doctors and nurses. And others in attendance who care about you — family and friends.

I always heal ahead of schedule due in part to my abstinence from pharmaceutical painkillers. I can't cite scientific studies to bolster my assertion, because such studies don't exist. We do know that all drugs pose risks, and all drugs produce unintended side effects. So if you can take the pain, don't take the painkiller.

Such a credo, "Take the Pain," has fostered my acceptance of paraplegia generally. After thirteen years of it, I indeed should accept my paraplegia. But I was just as okay with it after thirteen days. Friends describe my attitude as stoic acceptance or Buddhist detachment. I describe it as just me.

Thousands every year sustain SCIs. Someone seemed destined to occupy my bed in the rehab ward. It might as well have been me because I could take the pain. Next door to me, every night, and all night, a middle-aged woman wailed and wailed. "Why me?" was the gist of her wailing. While crossing the street, as though struck by lightning, she was nailed by a hit-and-run motorist. My attitude of "Why not me?" differed from hers because I had no one to blame but myself. No one pushed me off that footbridge. I dove of my own free will. Perhaps I've been in free fall ever since. The ride has been a wild and wide detour to my life that, if given the choice, I certainly would not have taken.

But given no choice, I endure paraplegia's detours and downturns. Children's stares and, what's worse, adults' averted glances. Flat tires and, worse, dog doo on fully inflated tires. Inaccessible public restrooms and, worse, no clean place to cath once inside the stall. The social stigma of being looked down upon for being crippled and, worse, the social isolation from being overlooked when you're seated at four feet tall. Not to mention the various health risks and complications, which I won't mention. Yet no matter how severe the humiliation nor deep the sorrow nor crippling the pain, I rest assured that after a good night's sleep, I'll get over it the next morning. "Take two aspirations and call me in the morning."

(Some object to the word "cripple." If I'm not "crippled," who the heck is? An "invalid" person and an "invalid" thing are the same word assigned different pronunciations and ascribed with different definitions. A person described as invalid thus can be associated as being a deficient object. It's politically correct to call an injured animal a cripple, so I side with the injured animal, in the same way I side with the scapegoat, the underdog, and the sitting duck.)

Occasionally I have achieved some lofty goals attainable only through paraplegia. Being very visibly crippled has some perks, and I've enlisted them to advance social causes.

Soon after my injury in 1990, I learned of an herbal remedy that both relaxes SCI spasms more effectively than tranquilizers and relieves SCI pains more safely than narcotics (not that I care about the pain). In 1996, in Europe, I procured a prescription for that herbal remedy from a Dutch physician. In January 1997, emboldened with my prescription and encouraged by recent referendums in California and Arizona, I wrote an editorial about my use of medicinal marijuana.

Connecticut's major newspaper, *The Hartford Courant*, displayed my public confession prominently and illustrated it very memorably. That single editorial garnered more reader response and more media attention than all my other books and articles combined. Since then, I've remained Connecticut's preeminent poster child for medicinal marijuana, which makes me half poster child and keeps me half flower child.

I accept full responsibility for my SCI. Society owes me nothing. I am able to stand on my own two feet. During all these years, I've lived independently, alone in a house in the woods. Those woods are part of a nature preserve where hunting is banned, but along whose shores duck hunting in the river was legal.

Before my injury, I participated in the outdoor sport of scaring away ducks from flying within range of shotguns. After rehab, I returned home in time to hear the shotgun blasts heralding duck hunting season. Seated in my wheelchair, I swore that next year I'd get out there to compete against the duck hunters again. And I did, but with crutches, and with one surprise. I was arrested for hunter harassment. The newspaper stories about my heinous crime could have been headlined, "Lone Cripple with Crutches Arrested for Harassing Four Hunters with Guns," but their titles were more diplomatic. The newspaper reports generated public support. Long dismayed about duck hunting on the shoreline of the nature preserve, advocates wrote letters, made phone calls, signed petitions, attended hearings. Our state legislator was enlisted, and state wildlife staffers made a field trip to the crime scene. By next season, the waterways along the nature preserve in which I live were banned to duck hunting.

A born-again pedestrian, I've resumed all my other previous vocations and avocations, including nature photography. The world I now photograph, however, has narrowed in focus. I photograph mostly my backyard. And sometimes, my front yard. One recurring theme is "Seasons in Sequence" in which I return to the same site during different times of day and on different days. Every year, I scout out and set up a new shoot spot. This enables me to view nature more clearly, or at least more comfortably. I clear a path so I can navigate in my wheelchair, or so I won't stumble with my crutches. I set up shop, and then just sit. I wait for birds to sing, or clouds to lift, or wind to settle, or thoughts to crystallize. Some evenings, I shoot the breeze. Many mornings, I shoot the sunrise.

"Deer Family Photos" is a recent theme. In 2001, I plotted to lure deer with food, and then to photograph them. Yet, if I simply appeared at my window from one hundred and fifty feet away, they'd spook and head for the hills. Slowly, slowly, I earned their trust. In early May, one very pregnant and very hungry doe lingered long enough for me to shoot the first of her family photos. By August, I could shoot her and her fawns from a hundred feet away. By October, fifty feet away. By spring 2002, I could shoot the yearlings from fifteen feet away. The peaceful evenings I share seated among the deer are more spiritually enriching than any other experience of my life. The endeavor needed much planning and patience. It also required approximately fifty bushels of cracked corn and exactly one wheelchair. The wheelchair is pivotal. Deer recognize me from a mile away. Seated, I'm their height, and so less intimidating. Indeed, I could not have entered into this communion afoot. I could attain it only in a wheelchair.

A wheelchair, however, hampers me elsewhere, for instance from access to the site of my injury. Yet I've managed to bridge that gap three times. People ask me, Why would I wish to return to a place of such bad memories? I instruct them that precisely by my being able to return, I transform my memory of that place into a good one. I crutched and, where necessary, crawled the steep one mile trail down to (and back up from!) that fateful footbridge. Because it was there. Because I wasn't. And because I may be crippled, but I ain't dead.

What's next? What's more challenging than being paraplegic for the rest of one's life? I suppose being paraplegic for the rest of one's life, and living to be a hundred. When I reach one hundred and one, then what? Dunno. I'll dive off that bridge when I come to it.

Mark Mathew Braunstein lives in Quaker Hill, Connecticut. He is an art librarian at Connecticut College, a widely published nature photographer, and author of two books and many articles about art, literature, philosophy, vegetarianism, and wildlife.

Never Should on Yourself

Renee Alper
C1-2
Age at SCI: 31
Date of SCI: February 23, 1989
Mason, Ohio

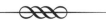

When I was 31, I was already leading a different life than most people, as I had developed a severe kind of arthritis thirteen years earlier and spent most of my time in a wheelchair. On February 23, 1989, I was traveling home from a day trip to visit my boyfriend in Columbus, Ohio, about two hours from my home in Cincinnati. We were driving slowly due to bad weather, but not slowly enough, apparently. We slid on the ice, and crashed off the side of the road. I hit my head, passed out, and when I woke up, I couldn't move, or even breathe. My friends were trying to move me, and I could not get any air through my lips to tell them not to. As they picked me up, it freed the blockage my vertebrae were causing in my spinal cord. I was then able to breathe and talk, but I had broken my neck in numerous places.

I was unable to move my left arm, I could not focus my eyes, and I had severe flexor spasms in my left leg, sometimes causing my entire body to spasm. I spent fourteen hours in the emergency room, where I was placed in a halo brace. My doctor said that if I did not show significant improvement in five days, he would have to operate on my neck, possibly causing total paralysis, or even death.

In the past, my father had divorced my mother because of my illness, and she had forbidden me to be seen outdoors by our neighbors because of her embarrassment at having a disabled child. At the time of the accident, both my parents were out of the countr, and were unable (or unwilling) to come see me.

I spent six months in a halo brace. During that time, when my boyfriend left me, I felt like the world had ended. I couldn't read, or even sit up for very long. I was bitter, crying to myself, "Not only am I trying to heal from a broken neck, I'm also trying to heal from a broken heart." Pity party was the word of the day.

Yet, it was in this state that I met my best friend Stan. He lived nearby, and had heard about my accident through mutual friends. At first, he brought his guitar over to entertain me, and then, as we became closer friends, he helped me overcome numerous obstacles along the path of healing. He increased my visual stimuli while in bed by putting up pictures that were changed regularly and developed better ways for people to move and position me, both in the chair and in bed. With his help, I learned to solve problems from new angles by reconstructing them in different ways.

I solved my problem with finding good live-in help by using two caregivers in a week, neither of them being a true live-in. This had seemed unstable and unsafe to me, but I overlapped their in and out times and hired people who wouldn't leave me until I was covered, trusting that I would continue to be safe. I have found that my attitude is almost always the part of a problem I can most easily change, and luckily, it is the thing I have the most control over.

Stan also taught me that no matter how terrible something I might have to face in the future seemed, if it wasn't happening to me right now, and if I'd already taken every possible step I could to safeguard myself against it, there was nothing to be gained by worrying about it and spoiling a perfectly good day — today. Tomorrow, and its possible problems, would come soon enough, and sometimes, I found, they never came at all.

After the brace was off, I began rebuilding my life. I did range of motion therapy with my friend Eric, a licensed medical massage therapist and medical student. Inspired by Eric's desire to help others, and by his insistence that there was a reason why I was here, I decided that my challenges needed to have meaning, and that meaning would come from teaching others. I thought of myself as having a mission to show others how much they had to be grateful for. But ultimately, it was because of all the blessings that I myself had that I found the path toward contentment.

One day, Eric asked me, "Do you know that you can be completely content even if nothing in your life improved from the way it is now?" I answered, "Sure, I know, on some esoteric level, that's true. They say that, given the right attitude, even a prisoner being tortured can find contentment. But come on, Eric, look at how my life is: incredible pain, stuck in a wheelchair with spasms, limited mobility, enormous problems finding personal care help — how can I be content?" He looked straight at me, and said, "Nevertheless, you can be completely content." I thought he was crazy, but a seed was planted that day. I realized that what he was saying was true, and it was up to me to find the way. It opened a door for me I would never have thought was there, just by believing that it might be.

I have learned that the first step toward changing anything is the belief that it can be changed. I was tired of people saying to me, "You have to look on the bright side of things. Count your blessings! Life is filled with abundance!" This seemed hopelessly unfair and inapplicable to someone who had as many problems as I. But what if they were right? So I tried it, and with practice, I found my life to be very, very rich, just by believing the richness was there.

Psychotherapy — with the right therapist — was an indispensable tool in my recovery. I have had excellent luck in this area, or perhaps it isn't luck at all. I shop for a therapist the same way I shop for a doctor. I explain that I am in charge of my care and am looking for specialists to be part of my medical team. I ultimately make the final and well-informed decisions for my body.

For the first time in my life, I am a habitual positive thinker. I never say, "I am..." anything that I don't really want to be, such as "I am so stupid," etc. I make sure I remember the positive attributes I have, even if other people have far more in some areas. There is always something else I could have lost and didn't. I try always to speak well to others, and if my pain and frustration cause me to speak poorly, I own my responsibility in that and try to make amends as soon as I am able. I look for "how to's," not excuses, such as trying to adapt an idea (or part of an idea) that someone has suggested, instead of finding fault with it. I can argue for my limitations and never change anything, or I can try to find a way to make something work and improve my situation.

I have become the teacher I wanted to be, but not because of how disabled I am, but how able I am despite my disabilities. I run my own personal care staff. I am a singer/songwriter, a public speaker, an actress/director, and a playwright. I have used my experiences to write a play about a disability support group, *Roll Model*, which recently had its world premiere.

I nurture myself when I can, by giving myself encouragement, praise, and sympathy, such as, "You're a good person; you don't deserve to hurt so much." I freely ask my friends to help nurture me when I can't do it for myself. I have learned that the secret to successful coping isn't about never falling down, but about always getting back up again. I have insight into the preciousness of life, even life with a spinal cord injury. Although some things in my body and my life are worse than they were at some points in the past, some things are better, and I celebrate them by reminding myself of this. I fill my days with productive activity and don't compare myself with where others are, or with where I could have been. And most of all, I forgive myself if I slip in any of these other things. "Never Should on Yourself" is my motto.

I thought, right after my spinal cord injury, that I would never be okay with eating out at a restaurant again. I didn't want people to stare at me as I was being fed (even with the arthritis, I had the ability to feed myself). But, as a character in my play says, "As long as you have a high profile, you might as well get some benefit from it." So, as a singer/songwriter, I do songs about disability, some happy, some serious.

I refer to myself as "the lady in the wheelchair with the dog." Both of my assistance dogs have been wonderful friends and terrific conversation starters. I don't worry much about what other people think of me. I'm fairly eccentric anyway, so my disability is just another quirk that makes me unique. I learned that having a spinal cord injury sucks, but letting it totally ruin your life sucks worse. I have also found that I have strengths I never imagined, and sometimes can't believe they come from the complaining girl I used to be. I can tolerate more pain, bounce back better from a bad day, and accomplish more than I ever thought I could.

My life is full. I live with my boyfriend, Ray, whom I met nine years after my injury. We sing together, and he helps take care of me. I go where I want when I can, and when I can't, I try to find some other positive thing to do. I am sad sometimes that I can't have much of what I would call physical fun (I loved swimming, biking, and miniature golf as a kid), but then, I chase my dog around the house with my chair, yelling "I'm gonna getcha!" at her (she loves it). It is good to be able to see, so I can drive my own chair. It is good to be able to hear, so I can listen to music and sing and go to the theatre. It is good to be able to speak, so I can communicate how I feel, and ask for the things I cannot do for myself. Most of all, it is good to be able to think, so I can make the best choices I can to make my daily living easier.

Some days I wonder if anyone who hasn't gone through what I've been through can understand the gifts that life has given them. I believe I am happier today than I would have been, had I not become disabled. This seems odd to me sometimes, but I remember being so unhappy when I was able-bodied that I know it must be true. But ultimately, it doesn't matter. I am here now, and where I would have been, no one will ever know. There is a Chinese philosophy known as "The Tao," which says life is a river. We can fight the current and tire ourselves trying, or we can "go with the flow," and use that current to further our journey to new places. Although I sometimes falter, most days, I am excited to be traveling my road and grateful for the friends who travel with me.

Renee Alper is originally from Chicago, but currently resides in Cincinnati, Ohio, with her significant other and her assistance dog, Star. Renee is a singer/songwriter, playwright, actress, director, and inspirational speaker. Other interests include holistic medicine, languages, computers, and the works of J.R.R. Tolkien.

No Roadblocks, Only Detours

David L. Baker
T5
Age at SCI: 45
Date of SCI: March 10, 1987
Essex, Maryland

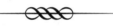

My life changed dramatically in March 1997. At 45, I suffered a descending dissecting aortic aneurism — "the big blood vessel coming from the heart, ripped open from the heart to the stomach." Surgery to repair the aneurism paralyzed me at the T5 level. I went from being a strong, active, outdoors person to a bedridden weakling. After several months of physical therapy, strong family support, and self-determination, I was able to enter the world again — but, it wasn't easy.

While I was in rehab, I could not believe that I had become disabled. I hated that word. I started to hate people who could walk, and even disabled people who were not as bad off as I was. I couldn't stand to think how I was going to be able to do all the things that I had done before. Sometimes, I even wished that I had not survived the surgery.

I had grown up in a loving and understanding family and was married to a loving and understanding wife. Although my wife and parents were very supportive, I did not perceive their words or actions as support. I was their son and husband; what else could they say besides, "Don't worry, everything will be okay"?

One event during rehab changed my thinking — and my life. I was sitting in the exercise room next to a lady with both legs amputated. She was about to receive her prostheses and was very excited. When she commented "I'm going to walk out of this hospital on my own two feet," I became so enraged inside that I had to return to my room. After sitting for a while, I began to think about how I had been. Why should I be upset at someone who was working as hard as she was to be able to walk again? After all, I wanted to walk again, too. Then I took a stroll around the floor and especially noticed people worse off than I was. I began to realize just how lucky I really was. Sure, there were people better off than me, but I had been raised not to be envious of others, and I was not going to let my disability change my values.

During childhood, I had several uncles who suffered from hip dysplasia, a genetic disorder carried by the women in our family that affects their male offspring and causes a missing limb or limbs, or a defect in a limb. I thought everyone had family members with defective or missing limbs. Uncle Ralph was born without legs. Growing up, I saw how Ralph coped. He drove a car, lived independently, and worked for the government in Washington. He lived a full life — all without ever complaining.

It was no big deal when I saw people using wheelchairs or crutches. I never treated anyone differently because of a physical condition. Coming from a family with a strong Christian background, I learned to accept people for who they are, not what they had or did not have — including physical abilities. I had grown up with my uncle and saw that his disability was more of a nuisance than anything else. Being disabled meant finding solutions to problems and not letting a problem beat you. I learned very early in life that no problem is too big, and every problem has a solution. I firmly believe that God will not challenge a person with more than he or she can handle. There are no roadblocks in life, only detours. Finding the right detour is the difference between accomplishment and failure. With all the disorders in my family, coupled with my faith, I believe I was better prepared to handle my disability.

I had been driving since I was sixteen and prided myself in being able to drive anything with wheels. Working at a local warehouse as a teenager, I had driven tractor-trailers. As an adult, I had a commercial driver's license and a rating to drive a motorcycle. I drove a heavy-duty rescue truck and an ambulance for a volunteer ambulance and rescue company. After my aneurism, I received a letter from the Motor Vehicle Administration stating that I had to surrender my license and take a test to be able to drive again. At first, I was angry. Then, realizing that not every paraplegic has the same motor skills or qualifications, I accepted the fact that I would have to demonstrate that I could still drive.

Since I had driven Uncle Ralph's car as a teenager, driving with hand controls was no big deal. I purchased a minivan with modifications that made it possible to drive from my power wheelchair rather than transferring from the wheelchair to the driver's seat. After driving around the neighborhood, the feel of the hand controls became second nature, and I felt ready to take my test. At the MVA, I surrendered my license and presented the letter to the clerk. Although I had driven my van less than twenty-five miles, I passed my test.

With my license and a van, I drove a few times with a passenger. I soon decided it was time to see just how independent I was. Since I had a lot of doctors' appointments following the surgery, I decided that I could go by myself and test my ability to maneuver the wheelchair and van without help. The first couple of doctor visits went fine and my confidence level was high. I felt that nothing could keep me down — until one day I went to a doctor's office where I had never been before.

I pulled into an accessible space in the parking lot where I could drop my ramp and disembark. After getting out, I noticed that I had forgotten to hang my "handicapped" placard on my mirror. Since I still had temporary tags on my van, I wanted to avoid any possible problems with the law by putting the tag where it belonged. Opening the side door and dropping the ramp, I started to enter the van when I felt my wheelchair start to flip over.

My sister had been telling me, that if I ever feel myself flipping over, to be sure to tuck my head forward and protect it with my arms so as not to bang it on the ground. In a split second, I went from going up the ramp to lying flat on my back, in the wheelchair, legs dangling above my head, looking up at the sky. Fortunately, I had protected my head.

After briefly looking up at the sky and making out different shapes from the clouds like I had done as a kid, I made sure I was okay and decided to get some help.

As a former first aid teacher who had always taught students to yell "Fire" in an emergency because it draws a crowd, I yelled "Help" one or two times. I was about to try "Fire" when a car pulled into the lot and, from the noise of the wheels, just missed my head. A couple got out and came to my rescue. I could tell that they too rode an ambulance or had training in first aid because their first words were, "Are you okay? Do you hurt anywhere?" As they began checking me, I explained that I was paralyzed and didn't have feeling where they were checking me — but that was normal for me.

Convinced I was fine, they set me and my wheelchair upright. I thanked them, asked the lady to put my placard on the mirror, and went on to my appointment. I told the nurse what had happened. After the visit, two nurses accompanied me to be sure I could get in without further mishaps. As I got into the van, we all laughed about my ordeal. I could have been irritated about what had happened, but laughing made it more bearable. I have learned to laugh more and get mad less. Getting mad doesn't solve anything. I now travel with a cell phone any time I am in the wheelchair, even if it's only to the front porch.

At home, things that I had done a million times before were now major milestones and learning experiences. One day, since the neighbors were gone for the day, I went next door to play with Bandit, a friendly golden retriever. Meanwhile, my wife had been making dinner and soon let me know that it was ready. As I started to leave, my wheelchair suddenly stopped moving — the batteries were dead. I had been riding around playing with Bandit, not watching my battery indicator. I grabbed my cell phone to call my wife, but it was dead too. I figured I would wait for her to come looking for me.

After about ten minutes, she did. The bad news was that I was downhill in my neighbors' grassy yard on a motorized wheelchair with a dead battery. The chair and I weighed about five hundred pounds and my wife had to push me uphill. By the time we got home, she was not talking to me very much. I promised to never leave the house without checking the batteries in the cell phone and the wheelchair and letting someone know where I was going. From all my experiences wheeling, I have learned to never assume anything and to expect the unexpected.

When I ventured out for a doctor visit after a snowstorm, I had a different learning experience. Knowing that the needed blood test would take several hours, I had decided that I would be fine by myself. After my appointment, I headed for the comfort of my nearby van. As I started up the ramp, I realized that there was snow on my wheelchair wheels. I kept spinning the tires causing my chair to go sideways, up the ramp — but only halfway up.

Eventually, a couple came walking by, and the young man asked if he could help. I instructed him to push on my knees as I applied power to the wheels. He was afraid of hurting me and asked if there was anywhere else he could push. After assuring him that he would not hurt me, we were able to get the wheelchair into the van. I learned that people are willing to help if asked, but can be afraid of hurting you and need to be assured that they will not — if they follow your instructions.

I am the same person today as I was prior to my injury seven years ago. My wife, Rita, has always been very supportive. Without her, I might have given up and ended my life. She and I found that the church and our faith in God helped us during my rehab and still continues to help us. I still enjoy talking with people and making new friends. I find that kids are curious about my wheelchair and how it works, but some adults are still leery of a person in a wheelchair.

I still try to learn something new every day just as I did before. I continue to learn about life as a normal person as well as life as a person with a disability. I am still learning that I can do things that I once thought I wouldn't be able to do — the latest example is going on a cruise. I feel much stronger and smarter than I was. In five years, I expect to know even more. I have never let anything beat me, and I will not start now.

David Baker lives in Essex, Maryland. On medical retirement from the phone company after twenty-five years of service, he has been married to Rita for twenty-nine years. He is a life member of the Middle River Volunteer Ambulance and Rescue Company, and continues to volunteer at area hospitals, working with SCI and sub-acute patients.

I Wasn't Born a Mermaid

Jaehn Clare
T12
Age at SCI: 20
Date of SCI: January 19, 1980
Atlanta, Georgia

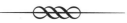

S urviving a spinal cord injury — a T12 incomplete compression fracture, resulting in paraplegia — taught me some noteworthy things.
First — I'm a survivor. A simple thing, but essential to my adaptation to life post-SCI. Knowing that I *am* a survivor puts me into quite a different relationship with adversity and mortality. Now I feel the truth of
Nietzsche's assertion "Whatever doesn't kill you makes you stronger."

Second — To sing out loud, even if with more enthusiasm than skill.
(For me it's mostly Jimmy Buffet, but Jackson Browne, Rickie Lee Jones,
Janis Joplin, and James Taylor will do it, too.)

Other inspiring tidbits include:
Let peace begin with me.
Approach cooking and loving with imagination and abandon.
Analyze capitalism; choose revolution; demand chocolate.
Forgive; floss; exercise — regularly.

Heed Goethe's advice:

> *Whatever you can do, or dream you can, begin it now.*
> *Boldness has genius, power, and magic in it.*

Five years post-SCI, I daydreamed that I might write a play about my experience. Ten years post-injury, I completed an original script as my master's project. The play premiered in 1990, in a seven-week tour of England and Scotland. On the eve of the fifteenth anniversary of my injury, I performed the play in Santa Barbara, California — a performance that later garnered an "Indie" award from the *Independent* newspaper. The process of writing and performing that play required that I face my fears, examining my injury and journey from the perspective of a storyteller. I was challenged to tell the story so that, as one early respondent noted, "One should care?"

[Sitting up slowly, Clarity slips the sheet off her legs, turning to face the audience, kneeling. Reaching up ...]

Clarity

I climb the ladder one step, one rung, one hand at a time. I reach the top. Over my left shoulder, the proscenium stage. To my immediate left, the two-hundred-fifty-seat auditorium. I see Tyler up in the catwalk, coiling a long snake of lighting cable. In my head, I hear the words "Good-bye, Tyler."

[Hands opening, lowering herself onto her haunches.]

This is bad! I'm falling; I'm going to hit the fl —

[Slaps her hands palm down, hard upon the floor, making a loud thud.]

OW!

[Slipping under the sheet.]

I lie supine. Immobile. Ambiguous. Surrounded by vast expanses of dim, white clinical odors. I sleep; I sleep — a lot. *[Suddenly fearful.]* Aaah! I'm awake. I'm not dreaming; not falling. I'm awake, I'm okay, I'm awake, I'm okay — okay, okay.

It took literally years, but eventually I was okay — I am okay. *Belle's on Wheels* — a semi-true story, mixing fact and fiction — helped shape my journey.

There is that immediate vulnerability post-injury — hurt, angry, scared, that broken place: "How the hell am I gonna do *this*?" From *there* to *here*. *Here:* a whole human life — working, loving, living — one day at a time.

Jessamyn

When you live inside a body labeled "disabled" you are defined as "Other"-than-human. It's not something people do on purpose — it just happens. This friend of mine says to me:

"I want to invite you to dinner, but I can't."

"Why not?"

"Well, there are stairs up to my house."

"So? I'll go up the stairs."

"But — you're disabled!"

"So? Will you help me?"

"Well, yeah."

"Great. When's dinner?"

I watch her face change as she tries to wrap her imagination around the image of me getting up a flight of stairs. She's having trouble envisioning exactly how I'll do it.

The writing began years before, during Recovery and Rehabilitation, with journaling; the first of several practices that alter my way of living. Others — reading, swimming, playfulness — also become part of "R and R." Among other things, I am required by my psychologist to examine how I allow other people's perceptions of me to shape my self-image. We talk about Fear — a lot. She shoves me right into the clutches of that cultural stigma associated with being "crippled."

R and R

[Clarity sits up briskly.]

Clarity

Recovery: the act or process of recovering. Recover: regain possession, use, control of; secure restitution or compensation; bring or come back to life, consciousness, health; retrieve, make up for, get over, cease to feel the effects of, make one's way back to ... Rehabilitate: restore normal capacities of disabled person, criminal, etc., by treatment or training; re-establish good reputation of, regain esteem for ...

I conscientiously journal on my emotional roller-coaster, noting my feelings and responses to people during daily life; the way I perceive other people's responses to me when I am doing the most mundane things like grocery shopping. Snatches of grassroots wit and wisdom — spiritual graffiti. Cultivating the habit of journaling pages and pages years before I ever hear about or see a copy of *The Artist's Way* by Julia Cameron or Natalie Goldberg's *Writing Down the Bones*, both of which influence my writing practice years later.

Page upon page, in more than thirty-five individual journals. I continue the practice, though not quite daily Morning Pages; sometimes it's afternoon, sometimes it's not pages — just little notes.

Live light, not lies.
Practice random acts of kindness & senseless acts of beauty.
I have enough; I do enough; I am enough!

I also still practice a little script I learned from that same therapist: "I refuse to be defeated by _____." And one fills in the blank. Fear. Apathy. Frustration. Others' narrow-mindedness. Lack of — anything. Money, self-esteem, energy. Some days it's simpler: "I refuse to be defeated." I decide; I'm not willing to fail because I didn't even try. It strikes me — I am not defeated because I am still willing to try.

The complement to the journal writing is a renewed interest in reading. As a twenty-something, in the first couple years of my recovery zone, I am gifted a copy of *The Tao of Pooh* by Benjamin Hoff. I lie in the grass literally all day long one Saturday — reading, chortling, giggling, laughing aloud, weeping, sighing. This gentle introduction to the classical Chinese text *The Tao Te Ch'ing*, and the Taoist principles of the complementary aspects of *yin* and *yang* deeply interest me. It provides just the sort of thing I need — a way to engage the effort to understand paradox and opposites.

Returning to my undergraduate studies feeds the need to read, and in completing my theatrical B.A., I also dabble in philosophy and the humanities. I read, work, perform here and there for years. At the second decade post-injury, I write a second play — *Tail Tell Tale,* a mermaid play — at my mother's urging.

Jessamyn

The Invisible Cripple Syndrome is brought sharply into focus at the reception for an art exhibit. We're all are dressed up, mixing, mingling, being seen. The guests walk around with their little plates balancing on their plastic wine cups. My little plate sits atop my wine cup, tucked between my knees. I patiently wind my way through the crowd. "Excuse me?," I ask a guest. "Pardon me. Excuse me, could I just sneak past you here?"

After three polite attempts, I am entitled to nudge him, just to give him a hint. So, I do — gently. He turns around, sees no one at his eye level, turns back to his conversation, stays right where he is. It takes me a minute to understand — this guy is just literally not seeing me. Suddenly, he turns in my direction, practically tumbling into my lap.

"Oops! Oh, sorry."

"It's okay. It's only a little red wine."

Then, right in front of me, I see the unexpected — another woman in a wheelchair. I greet her.

"Hello."

"Hi! How ya doin'?"

"Okay. Going slowly."

"Yeah. Me, too — it's a bitch, huh?"

"Yeah. I'm just trying to get to the bathroom."

"Try that way — the crowd's thinner down there."

"Thanks."

"Sure. Remember, after you run over their toes, they move."

Flashing me a broad grin, she wheels off in the direction of the bar, dodging the vertical guests deftly. I feel a small surge of satisfaction — I am not alone. I don't see her for the rest of the evening, but I feel better just knowing she's here — bumping legs, running over toes. Just knowing that she is somewhere in the room alters the whole event for me. We see each other. The other guests may not acknowledge us, but they can't make us invisible to each other. No one can make me invisible.

I give myself permission to explore my physical-ness as it is, reconfigured post-SCI. Sometimes getting around is tough, and I have injured myself more than once, but I want to be able to go out and about, living in the world, rather than cooped up, "shut-in." Experimentation taught what I can — and still want — to do. I have basically given up bicycling, which I did love. But I reclaimed swimming for myself. I allow my Self water-play-full-ness, and there comes with it a curious, strangely physical sensation of, "Hey! I'm still in here!"

Jessamyn

I can still swim. *[She slips off her wheelchair onto the floor.]* In the water, I let go. I move more readily and independently. I swim as physical therapy — a cardiovascular workout, aerobic conditioning, stamina building. I find much more than just physical strength in the water. It's a skin thang, too — the sensation of being touched all over my body, simultaneously. Touch deprivation is all-too-often accepted as a fact of life-with-disability. But when the water touches my skin, it reminds me — I need to learn to live in my skin again. Mermaids do! They live in their skins, without shame or embarrassment that they don't walk. How do I learn to live in such a way?

I get fed up with feeling pissed off *all* the time, so I make a vow to teach myself to have fun again. I start by enjoying — savoring — the simplest things. Looooong hot bubble baths; something not recommended for those wearing a cast, so I missed out on nine months of heavenly hot water. I'm still making up for lost bubble-time! And in honoring the vow to re-learn fun, I sometimes sang to myself in the bathtub. Oddly, it was learning to sing Jimmy Buffet out loud that conjured up the solution to my early existential crisis:

"I'd rather die while I'm living than live while I'm dead."

The swimming is something I enjoy doing without the wheelchair — and it has restored me to a fundamentally positive sense of my physical self. I also now do Pilates (floor exercises) without the use of the wheelchair. Even after twenty-three plus years, it's still a daily choice to feel good about my body. This body, the one I live in now.

A colleague once asked, "Do you consider yourself an artist, a woman artist, or a disabled artist?" My immediate response is, "Which day? What time?" I am a theatre artist; woman; person with a disability. None of these qualities encompasses the sum of my being; yet each expresses something true about me. And Survivor; I didn't know that prior to my injury. I do now; I value that. I'm not saying I would have chosen spinal cord injury as a path to personal growth, but the depth it has brought to my life is undeniable. After all the pondering, praying, reading, therapy, weeping, whining, blah-blah-blah — one day I bite into a strawberry, and I get it: Utter certainty that this Life is no accident. My injury may have been an accident — but that strawberry is no accident! And I believe that living is something I can do from the seat of a wheelchair.

Jessamyn

I wasn't born a mermaid. I evolved. It was a dramatic moment, not quite a fall from grace, but a fall nonetheless. But then, that's another story. This is a tale of a different sort, a transformative tale — transformation not of the outside-in, but of the inside-out.

Jaehn Clare lives in Atlanta, Georgia, with her partner Earl Daniels, his teenage daughter, two dogs and a cat. She is employed part-time as the Arts Outreach Coordinator at VSA arts of Georgia, and she freelances as a solo performer and teaching artist. Learn more about Jaehn at: www.JaehnClare.net.

Give It a Year

Steve Dalton
T4
Age at SCI: 34
Date of SCI: March 9, 2002
Novato, California

———————— ∞∞∞ ————————

*I*t's been a little more than a year since my paralyzing motorcycle accident. I was motorcycling in the eastern hills of the San Francisco Bay Area with a close friend and three of his buddies. I was leading on a road that I had only been on a few times. I got into a corner too fast, went wide, ran off the edge of the pavement onto the gravel, hit a small earth-berm protecting a drainage ditch, and was ejected on to the rocky hillside.

As I lay on the ground, I immediately knew I had sustained a spinal cord injury. I had spent six years as a motorcycle road racing track safety crew member, so I knew how to evaluate the situation. I knew the procedures for minimizing the trauma.

I first took inventory. Flex fingers: "Fingers, check." Flex wrists: "Wrists, check." Then, I got to my lower body. I couldn't move anything. I told my friends not to move me, not to take off any of my gear. When the volunteer fire department arrived forty minutes later, I continued to direct things, giving them my symptoms, telling them to cut off my expensive riding gear. Twenty minutes later, I was on a chopper, in good hands, and free to drift into unconsciousness.

The most serious injury was trauma to my spinal cord from the crushed vertebra at T4. Four days after my accident, I underwent surgery to fuse the T2 - T8 vertebrae. The Santa Clara Valley Medical Center team came out of surgery very optimistic about the success of the procedure, especially that the fracture at C7 would not impact the cord.

My first week in the hospital was very busy — and morphine filtered. Family and friends filed in and out continuously. We talked a lot, cried some, and even laughed — allowing ourselves some black humor. I maintained a positive outlook, confident that everyone around me was doing their best. I relaxed, and accepted that this was a process I would not be able to rush. It My attitude helped me. It helped all of those around me.

Four nights after surgery, I lay awake in bed and began to cry. My body wasn't telling me that I'd walk again. I sobbed for an hour. I didn't really examine it closely at the time, but now I know it was a mixture of feelings. I didn't want to disappoint my family and friends, who were all so confident that I'd be "up and walking around in no time." I knew this was my wife Tracy's worst nightmare — a disabling injury from riding. And I was simply scared; I didn't know what this would mean in my life. I didn't tell anyone about this night for almost two months.

Ten days after my injury, I was transferred into the rehab unit. The nurses and physical therapy staff assured me that I was ready, saying, "You've come so far since surgery. Look how long you've stayed up in your wheelchair after just two days."

I wasn't so sure. I like to know what to expect, but I had no idea what rehab was going to be like. The staff had started training me right away in the hospital, but there was so much to absorb. It was an intimidating scenario, so I didn't ask all the questions I might have. And I was still scared.

Rehab was tough. The therapists assured me I'd do well: "You've got full use of your arms and most of your chest. You're totally going to be able to take care of yourself when you're released." But I struggled learning to dress myself independently. By the time I went home, I had still never gotten myself off the floor into my chair unassisted. Other patients were doing these things. I should be able to figure this stuff out! I had always been pretty athletic. Why was it so difficult for me to master these tasks? I later realized that each SCI patient has different outcomes, and I shouldn't compare myself to others.

I found tremendous encouragement in all of the calls, cards, and visits from family, friends, and co-workers. Everybody was rallying around me. It felt good. I knew it was because I was staying positive. I didn't know if they would stick with me if I let myself get down. I thrived on their approval.

There were plenty of breakthroughs. I made an effort every day to look at even the smallest achievements. I made a point to talk to my friends and family about what I accomplished that day that I hadn't done before. This helped me build on my successes.

There were peer support group meetings in rehab, where my internal doubts competed with my optimism. Initially, I thought skeptically, "Peer support, whoopee!" I expected a psychologist encouraging us to "talk it out." Former patients often participated. One night, we heard from three who were two to four years post injury. They were all working, driving, and living independent lives. They said, "Everything changed in the first year after my injury," and "You won't believe where you'll be in a year." They were referring not only to how their bodies changed, but how they adjusted psychologically to living with SCI. It gave me what I needed — a sense of what to expect. I was still very scared, but the support groups helped me see that I could be okay.

My inpatient peers were coping with their injuries in different ways. Some were more scared and lost than I was. For most of rehab, my roommate was angry, demanding attention from the staff and not actively participating in his rehab. Others kept at it even though they struggled with some of the activities. I was surprised to find that my example — keeping a positive attitude and going with the process — seemed to encourage and inspire some of the others around me to work harder. It was an unexpected reward.

Some of the hardest times were emotional, not physical. Like when I finally told people I didn't believe I'd walk again. I told my wife, Tracy, and my best friend, Brad. They were both crushed to hear me express that doubt, but they reacted differently.

Brad responded with love and grief. He heard what he did not want to admit. We both worked through the sorrow of that moment. Tracy responded with anger, accusing me of giving up while everyone around me stayed positive. I didn't know how to deal with her reaction.

While I'd been physically injured, the emotional injury was much more far reaching. My friends, family, and most of all, my wife, were affected by their own emotions surrounding my accident. Tracy, especially, struggled with this nightmare that had become real.

She and I had been having difficulty communicating even before the accident. My accident intensified the issues for us. It's a three to four hour round-trip from our home to the hospital. So we talked mostly by phone. As often as we had warm supportive conversations, we had heated disagreements. When she was at the hospital, she didn't like coming to the rehab sessions, saying she couldn't stand seeing me have to work so hard at things that used to be so easy. These interactions hurt. It felt like she was withdrawing.

I sometimes resented the emotional turmoil in our relationship. I found myself conflicted, wanting to reach out to her, but also angry. I was the one in the hospital, I needed support. I wanted to focus on my recovery, not navigate a minefield of emotions.

As we prepared for discharge, there were some other challenges ahead. We live in a two-story house where I couldn't get into any of the bedrooms or bathrooms. I couldn't yet do my bowel program alone. We had planned on my mom helping with that — Tracy couldn't do it because of a neck problem. But Mom wouldn't be in the area until ten days after release. My insurance was refusing to pay for a homecare nurse. How were we going to deal with this?

I worked with my case manager to get a nurse approved for the first ten days. Tracy set up a bed downstairs and made a place in the laundry room for a tub bench where I could do my bowel program. Taking action helped us overcome the anxiety associated with the obstacles.

Home. Now came the test to see if I could apply my newly learned skills without the safety net of therapists and nurses. Everything looked like it was going to work just fine. I was happy and feeling confident. But Tracy was incredibly protective of me. Since she hadn't been able to see much of my physical therapy, she didn't have the reassurance of knowing what my level of skill was. She worried about every transfer, every trip in and out of the house. She felt our home had become a prison for me.

We still struggled with the emotional trauma. Tracy had predicted this would happen, in an argument four years earlier. "What will happen when you get hurt?! Will your riding buddies come take care of you? No, I'll be stuck with it!" She felt burdened by the care I needed, but also felt compelled to give it. I vehemently disagreed with that perception. I contended that I could do more to help, but she didn't agree. We both wanted to regain control of our lives. This initial period was incredibly frustrating for me. We've both learned to loosen our grip, and we continue to look for balance and mutual respect.

After getting home, I began outpatient physical therapy, where I achieved the floor-to-wheelchair transfer. I improved my mobility, mastering wheelies and jumping curbs. I found a gym where I could work out. My successes in therapy and at the gym have made a really positive difference in my self-perception.

I began to rebuild my life. I've found that when my friends and family see me, they lose this stereotypical vision of a frail, fragile, attendant-laden, and sterile invalid, and see a healthy Steve who uses a wheelchair for mobility.

I've returned to work in a technical support position for a nonprofit land conservation group, gradually working back to full-time status. I've since been promoted. I've found organizations that have enabled me to go kayaking, water-skiing, and downhill mountain biking.

I've also returned to the racetrack to stay connected to my passion for motorcycle racing and my friends there. I've worked on a safety crew this year. I wondered if I'd still be able to do it, so I had to try. I almost turned around while driving to the track. I found I could still do it — and enjoy it. I had reclaimed another portion of my life.

I continue to see a neuropsychologist who has helped me sort out my feelings about the injury and the changes in my life, my marriage, my self-image. Tracy and I continue to work on our relationship, though she is uncomfortable with participating in counseling together. We're still struggling for control, for ways to feel empowered. I remain optimistic that our life can be joyful and rewarding, and believe we can share that together.

This year has not been easy, but it's been rewarding. I'm healthy, in great shape, I have mastery over my daily activities, I lead an active lifestyle, I'm independent, and I'm committed to progressing further. I've learned that I am much more capable than I thought. I honestly feel more self-confident now than I ever have before. I expect that next year will be even better.

Steve Dalton lives in Novato, California. He works as a network support specialist for The Trust for Public Land. He enjoys music and outdoor recreational activities, and continues to learn and share with others the experience of living with SCI.

My Rides in Hearses

Walter Kimes
C5-6
Age at SCI: 20
Date of SCI: October 15, 1955
Sandy Lake, Pennsylvania

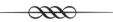

*H*aving been told several times over the years by various doctors that I have survived being a high level traumatic quad as long as anyone east of the Mississippi River, I often wonder how and why that came to be. I am well aware that part of the answers is good luck, much more than good management, at least where my efforts were concerned. Back in 1955 when I became a C5-6 quad in a car accident, very few people with broken necks survived beyond a few months or so. Due to a lack of precedent, medical care for quads was comparatively primitive and experimental.

Three of us guys were riding in the front seat of a new, 1956 Ford Crown Victoria. I was twenty years old, and sitting in the middle "suicide" seat. All three of us were thrown out of the car when the doors were torn off as it turned over sideways and end over end several times. There were no seat belts in cars back then. We landed in a swampy area, and the car came down right side up on top of the driver where the red-hot dual exhausts

burned him badly and fractured a few bones also. The third passenger suffered only a scratch on one ear.

Shortly after my accident, I still vividly recall coming to, in no pain
but unable to move anything below my neck. I heard the blood curdling
screams of the car's owner/driver and then saw this nifty-looking maroon
1940 Cadillac La Salle hearse pull up nearby. In my area of rural Western
Pennsylvania, there were no ambulances then. The local funeral director and
his hearse served double duty as hearse and as an ambulance, as needed. I
thought, "Shit! I really did it this time!"

The small country hospital I was taken to at first had a difficult time
trying to figure out what was the matter with me. After several hours, they
sent me to a bigger hospital about fifty-five miles away in a 1953 Cadillac
hearse that had a flat tire midway on the trip, at 3 a.m. My dad rode along
in the hearse, and he held cigarettes for me as I drifted in and out of awareness. No oxygen or EMTs in a hearse to say, "No Smoking."

The next thing I recall was waking up about three weeks later, then
drifting in and out of awareness for another week or two. I was like a piece
of sandwich meat between two slices of bread. The bread was two canvas
stretchers, with the bottom one having a hole in it for my backside, and
the other one having two holes in it: one for my face and one for my pri-
vates. I was held in place by three bed sheets wrapped around me. One
around my face, one around my waist, and one around my ankles. In this
contraption, I was turned every two hours, 24 hours a day. It took three
people to turn me each time. It was called a "Stryker frame," but I called
it much worse — and quite often, too.

Two holes were drilled in each side of my head, where ice-tongs were
clamped and attached to about eighteen pounds of weights to immobilize
my head and neck, even while turning me over. I also had a tracheotomy in
my throat, several IVs in my arms and a blankety-blank catheter to urinate.
I must have been a gruesome sight to behold, with my shaved head and ice-
tongs, iodine and bandages everywhere, and tubes galore.

No one would let me see a mirror, despite my repeated requests and
pleas, nor would anyone hold a cigarette for me. I went from 165 down to

100 pounds in just several months, and was somehow aware that I looked and smelled like a mess.

Daily enemas did not help my attitude one bit. I was a miserable, impatient, very scared and profane patient. I couldn't use my arms at all, so I had to be hand-fed — even though I found out later that I could, but I just didn't give a shit enough to even try. For the first year, I had private-duty, around-the-clock nurses, and I was rather hard on all of them. And on my very supportive family.

At first, the doctors vaguely implied that I likely would "be up and around" again in a few more months or so, and that gave me some hope, which I magnified beyond reason for the first eight or ten months. Then, I slowly came to realize how dumb I was to ever believe any doctor or nurse. I was kept in the hospital for five years. I must have been in denial up to then, but then deep depression set in, and I thought I was losing my marbles.

I became obsessed and preoccupied with suicide and how in hell could I do it with absolutely no movement below my neck. For many an hour those were my sole thoughts and, of course, it was all very frustrating to me.

Numerous urinary and respiratory infections pushed me deeper into my funk. I slept or pretended to sleep much of the time to shut the real world out and to have more time to dwell on my morbid thoughts — even after I got out of the Stryker frame and into a normal hospital bed. They still had to turn me over every two hours. I became an expert at getting sleeping and pain pills from the doctors and nurses.

Back in those days of four beds to a room, they had strict 2:00 to 4:00 and 7:00 to 9:00 p.m. visiting hours by family only. But I had a private room and could have any visitor, any time. My mom came to see me every day from about 11 a.m. until 10:30 at night. She kept me, somehow, from going completely around the bend. I was always a good reader and liked stories, so she read to me a lot from newspapers, books, and some magazines. Frequent visits from my sister and dad were also a huge help. I sorely needed all of them to help me keep in touch with reality.

The hospital kitchen made whatever I wanted to eat and all the hospital staff generally spoiled me. I had a pretty good appetite, though for some reason I still lost quite a bit of weight. After I was there for about three years I got a TV, the first one in the whole hospital, and still the only one when I left after five years. Despite all of these perks, privileges, and support, I was still deep into my own private pity party and a nasty S.O.B. to everyone in sight.

I wondered for a long time why no one ever tried to figure out if I could use my arms, but I guess they just didn't expect anyone with a broken neck to live. I was probably the first one that ever did in this particular small town area. I did start to wonder why the doctors didn't ask some questions or tell me to wake up and smell the roses or some damn thing, but I got no answers. But I never asked them either.

Then, the first physical rehabilitation center in Western Pennsylvania opened, St. Francis Hospital in Pittsburgh, and my old family doctor somehow got me in there — the second patient they admitted. Fortunately, it was a new wing to an existing hospital, and after an alcohol wash of my spine, removal of my right kidney and intense treatments of my bed sores, the occupational and physical therapists were able to get my arms to move, enable me to sit up in my very own, first-ever wheelchair, smoke my own cigarettes, and even to feed myself — sort of anyway.

At first I couldn't tolerate sitting up for more than a couple of hours at a time. Before, I didn't have any motivation to do anything, so I didn't. At the rehab hospital I saw what other quads could do, and I wanted to be like them, so I got motivated. I had some psychiatric counseling, too, for half an hour a day for the better part of a year.

By making this huge progress and being around others much worse off than I thought I was — quads who had brain damage or higher injuries and never made any progress while I was there — my mental state improved considerably. After getting sideways drunk with my three roommates a few times, it slowly dawned on me that just maybe life wasn't a complete bummer after all.

After more than seven months in the physical rehabilitation center, I was transferred to a first and fairly new physical and vocational rehab center in Johnstown, Pennsylvania. After constant problems with bed sores, I was sent home after twenty-one months. After nearly eight years post-trauma, I finally got to go home for the first time. I thought it was just for one day, that I was going to have to go to a nursing home, and that they just did it as a change of pace or a morale booster I guess. It was my birthday, too. I wasn't expected to go home and stay home. But the County Poor Farm was our closest thing to a nursing home then, and my family ruled that out as an option. Thank goodness.

My dad was a saint for taking care of me for years once I was back home. He had a full-time job and did it all by himself because my mom had died while I was in the rehab center. He later remarried.

By this time, my mental state had vastly improved. Even though I was now able to commit suicide, I no longer wanted to. Slowly, almost unnoticed by me, somewhere along those eight years, I became damn near normal once again. Whatever "normal" may be to each of us.

The passage of time, contact with other gimps, lots of very nice and helpful people, the one hundred percent support of my family and a new awareness of the constant beauty around us — sunrises, sunsets, play of muscles in a helpers arms and legs, causing someone to smile, an antique car, smells of supper cooking, looking ahead to some event — all of these were invaluable to me and still are.

At my advanced age of 68, I've given up hope of crossing paths with a soul mate and having a family, but in the back of my mind it's still there a little bit.

Since 1970, I have been self-employed at home, preparing income tax returns, as a Notary Public, issuing boat licenses, and doing bookkeeping for small, local businesses. Since my dad died in 1988, I live alone and have helpers who come in three times a day to give me a big hand.

Life is worth living, and I regret the fact that it took me so many years to realize that fact. I still very much resent the fact that I am not able to be up and about, have my own family, and leave my mark on the world. But, in a way that I can't explain even now, I can now accept these facts without having another pity party over them. I reckon even pity parties get boring after a while — whether drunk or sober. I think there is something to the old cliché that goes something like: "Surviving the bad times makes one more appreciative of the good times. Beauty surrounds us, but it's up to us to notice it and to enjoy it. All it costs is giving up some self-absorption, so the price is right, too."

Afterthought: Can't sleep? Try counting your blessings.

Walter Kimes lives in Sandy Lake, Pennsylvania, the same area where he was born and raised since 1935. He lives alone thanks to the able support of aides who assist him three times per day. He is self-employed and works from his home.

August

Kimberly Clarke
C5-6
Age at SCI: 17
Date of SCI: August 27, 1997
Setauket, New York

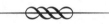

*I*t's not just the hot, humid, uncomfortable New York weather that makes me a crazy person every August. It's the three and a half weeks building up to August 27 that gets my panties all in a bunch. August 27 is the day my whole life changed — a 180-degree flip into a hell I never knew existed. I felt like I went from the age of seventeen to thirty in a split second — and became jaded for the rest of my life.

At first, I wasn't jaded; I was overly optimistic — I would go back to life as usual, attend my senior prom, and go off to college. I was optimistic that I would walk in time for my "adult" life to start. I was seventeen and had no clue how breaking my neck would change my life.

Six years later, I'm still finding out. It is like being in a huge maze. Every time I come to a corner there's more to the maze and big, huge monsters potentially lurking around each corner. These monsters don't have faces to scream at or bodies to beat on. Instead, they are infections that beat me up or frustrations like failing my driving test repeatedly because the equipment is so high tech and overwhelming that I lose my confidence behind the wheel. They can also be the embarrassment of bladder or bowel incontinence or the disappointment of being unable to attend a function with a loved one because of inaccessibility.

When I meet new people, I can tell that they are anxious to find out what type of horrible accident put me in a wheelchair. It's almost like they have this list in their heads that contains activities that should never be attempted because they could kill, paralyze, or maim. So when people hear my story, they get freaked out because lots of people have ridden a horse. It's not an unreasonable pastime.

Like most teenagers at seventeen, I thought I was hot shit. While visiting my grandparents and aunt in North Carolina, I was eager to ride my aunt's horse. I was a moderately experienced rider and felt secure in my abilities. All that stands out in my memory about that day is eating tuna fish and grapes, the almost unbearable heat that felt like it was piercing through to my insides, the amazing exhilaration of the freedom I felt riding a horse, and the fear as I was suddenly lying on the ground unable to move.

I didn't grasp what had happened to me. I don't really remember any one person telling me straight out that I had broken my neck. I'm sure that someone, probably a lot of people, at some point explained to me what I had done and the severity of my situation. I simply do not remember. That's how the next three months were — I do not remember.

I have heard some people describe themselves as the same person except without the ability to walk. While that may be true for some, I cannot whole-heartedly believe that a person who has been faced with even temporary paralysis comes through unchanged and unscathed. It's not just losing the ability to walk, but also the ability to move. I, as a quadriplegic, have probably lost the ability to move more than two-thirds of my body's muscles. Lying on my back, I can't sit up or even roll onto my side. That's what I have had to adapt to — and more.

Along with the physical aspects of SCI, there are the mental/emotional aspects. In my opinion, there were two ways to deal with my injury. I could choose to either live or die. Sometimes, it got so bad that I had to make that decision on a daily — or even hourly — basis. There have been many times in the past six years when I simply asked myself if it is worth it.

I remember my high school graduation. Everyone convinced me to take part and, for some reason, I agreed. My best friend offered to wheel me up to accept my diploma and everything went smoothly. All I could think about, though, was whether living was worth all these people seeing how helpless I had become. Now, I know that it is.

Someone once told me that the only reason he was still alive is because he couldn't open the bottle of pills. After his confession, I vowed to myself that I would never do that. I reasoned that if I chose to die, that was it — no going back. But, if I chose to live, life always had that potential to get better, to "right" itself.

Making the decision to keep on living was surprisingly easy while I was in rehab. Everyone around me seemed so positive. I believed I was supposed to focus on getting better and start putting my accident behind me. No one ever said that to me out loud, but I felt that these were the secret wishes of my family and friends. I obliged without question. I felt that if my family and friends could see my pain, they would be in so much more pain. I knew that my accident had already caused them so much grief that I felt obligated to move on with my life so they could move on with theirs.

Being seventeen, I didn't understand how this would affect my life when I got discharged from the hospital. I was very ambitious and thought I'd do everything I planned on doing during my senior year. On my first day back at school, I arrived in a little yellow school bus, four periods late, and making a scene on a very noisy wheelchair lift. I knew I wasn't going back for a second day.

It was a defining moment for me. I made the decision not to go back to high school out of pure fear. I was so afraid of being different — normal for a teenager. Going back that day put my biggest fear into reality. Every moment, I was aware of how different I was and how, no matter how hard I tried, I couldn't escape the things that made me different — my wheelchair, the noisy lift, and the woman pushing me around.

That's when things truly started to change. I knew I wasn't going to go back to school, attend my senior prom, or go back to life as usual. In one split second, I lost that life. I grieved for that life for a very long time. My grieving was most poignant while I watched my friends do stuff I would have done with them if it weren't for my paralysis — camping out on the beach, hiking upstate, or attending two-day Phish concerts. I smiled and listened to their adventures quietly as I felt this hole in my heart throb. Today, six years later, I still grieve at times.

I never cried to my friends about missing out on activities with them. I hid my grief from them as much as I could because my emotional pain was so intense that I didn't want them to feel even a bit of it. Until my paralysis, I never knew what heartache was. My heart physically hurt as I wept for my former life when I was alone. To this day, I cannot bring myself to share my deepest pain regarding my injury. Only I know how much it hurts.

After my injury, I believed I would just blend back into the life I led before. But, the life I led and the person I was before are completely different than the person I am becoming and the life I am leading now. I wonder, sometimes, if a part of me is still in denial.

Dealing with my SCI has been very hard on my mind. I can't begin to count the times I have woken to find that what I thought I was dreaming was, in fact, the life I was living. There was nothing scary about what I dreamt. It only turned into a nightmare after I woke up, realizing I can't get away from my SCI — even in my dreams. Being in that moment when I'm not fully awake is like a huge tease because, for a split second, I feel relieved it was a dream. When that moment fades, I am faced with the excruciating disappointment that I cannot move and what I prayed was a dream is actually my life.

SCI also killed a piece of my heart. I always took for granted that I would be able to play tag with my future children, walk my dog, or even just feed myself. I use the word kill because that piece of my heart will never come back; there is always a scar. I believe, though, that a new piece slowly grows over the old piece and appreciates what I can do. I can express my love for my family and friends and am learning to live on my own independently.

What I can do now, six years post, is leaps and bounds more than I could do at the beginning of my injury, or even one or two years ago. Most recently, I finally was able to catheterize myself. This is a huge accomplishment in my fight for my independence. It allows me to be able to rely more on myself than others and makes my dream of living on my own more feasible.

Living on my own is my goal. Right now, I attend community college. After I finish, I hope to transfer to a university in California. I think I have finally figured out what I would like to do with my life. Social and advocacy work are two of my main interests. I plan on getting degrees in social work and law so I can help people make a better life for themselves. I realize I will never be rich doing such work. There is one good thing that has come out of my injury — my priorities are in better order now. I value relationships more than possessions and appreciate the feeling of being content with what I have.

One relationship, in particular, has been a major catalyst in my changing of priorities. I guess falling in love will do that. I had never been in love before and couldn't fathom, disabled or not, that I could find someone I have so much chemistry with and who makes me feel so accepted. When we got involved I never expected to get what I got. I never expected to fall as hard as I have, and I certainly never expected someone to love me as much as he does. He deals with my SCI issues with grace and helps me feel the least disabled when I am with him. Our relationship has helped shift my priorities because looking at him makes me realize that no possession could make me as happy as being with him does and that no stress, SCI related or not, is as important as loving him is. The great part about this relationship is that he is so much more than a guy that I'm in love with. He's a great friend — a person that gives me a reason to keep moving forward in life even when I feel like I can't — and a soul mate.

"Dealing with" an SCI is not something that runs its course, moves on, and then we're fine. It's an everyday struggle. As I move on in life, I believe it becomes more of a private, personal battle. I know I rarely let my family or friends in on my "tough quad days." Those are the days that kick my ass and make me feel like I'm drowning. On the days I do let my family or friends in, I call on the few that calm my soul and let me be crazy or quiet without judging or wondering why. These people — childhood girl friends and my special guy friend — are the people I cherish. I let them in, and they help me by bringing laughter into my day. They help me believe I still fit in somewhere, even if I feel very displaced from the norm because of my disability. I think, for the most part, I have claimed my disability for my own and realize that I'm the only one "dealing" with an SCI. They just watch.

Kimberly Clarke lives in Setauket, New York. She is a college student living with her family. She is majoring in social work and is an aspiring writer.

The Water's Just Fine

Gary Karp
T12/L1
Age at SCI: 18
Date of SCI: July 4, 1973
San Rafael, California

T here was only time to respond from instinct, spreading my arms as I fell to keep my balance. It felt like I'd landed flat on my back, but my friends who had the horror of witnessing it say that I landed on my butt first. That explains why my back broke at T12/L1, where the bottom ribs meet — and so reinforce — the spine. I was instantly unable to move my legs.

There had been a major storm in Southfield, Michigan, where I grew up. A neighbor had hired us to clear his property. One tree needed to be cut down, so, on the morning of the Fourth of July, having never handled a chain saw in my eighteen years of life, I stood twenty-five feet up without a belt, about to sink the blade into a large upper branch that had to be trimmed off first. I had barely cut into it when the branch broke of its own weight, the tree shifted violently, and now I have a frozen memory of that moment in the air, aware I was falling.

There was a huge outpouring of support from my family and friends during the subsequent hospital stay — basically a nonstop gift- and food-laden party. Following five hours of surgery to rebuild my spine, I had woken up in a circle bed — a Ferris wheel kind of thing, with the bed as the diameter. It was used to rotate me between back and belly to prevent pressure sores. We performed the operation every four hours, day and night, for six weeks.

I expected to recover. No one claimed anything to the contrary, except my orthopedic surgeon, who, in answer to my asking how long it would be before I could be back on the ski slopes, suggested I deal with first things first. I was left to operate on the assumption that I would recover. Part of me knew better.

I was at last getting what I'd been craving all my life (with the brief exception of my Bar Mitzvah) — being the center of attention. The baby of three boys, I envied my big brothers their privileges. So, I played right into being the young hero, basking in the waves of approval for my spirited, positive response to my injury.

At the Detroit Rehabilitation Center, the assumption was that I was going to work hard and be independent. The weightlifting was so intense that to this day I have stretch marks on my shoulders. The skin couldn't keep up with the expansion of my muscles.

A rehab social worker surprised me saying, "We're all waiting for you to get depressed." That wasn't my style. My approval-seeking habit didn't allow for being openly sad or angry. It's not an effective way to get people to like you. Besides, I felt good about myself for the way I was succeeding at the work of rehab.

Seven weeks later — thirteen after the injury — well-trained for life using wheels, I came home to the news that, the day before, my father was found in his car on the side of the road, dead of a heart attack. He was en route to his new drugstore, due to open in two weeks. The year before he had sold the store he owned for twenty-five years in a working-class neighborhood where he was honored as a friend and advisor. I had worked there since I was eight, absorbing my father's charismatic, strong example.

I barely grieved. It was another event to just take in, to move through. I was too deeply in the mode of getting back into the world and too emotionally protected to even feel the full impact of the news. Denial was undeniably my main coping mechanism.

I also adapted by doing — getting back on the road with hand controls, going to outpatient therapy, starting architectural school, having missed only the fall term, and renewing my efforts to find the love of my life. I just got myself out there, thinking of it as being like jumping off of a diving board into cold water; the trick was to get yourself in the air, then you have no choice but to adjust.

My disability identity felt foreign. In public, in my mind, I would think to the people around me, "But I'm one of you! I was walking just a few months ago!" I was uncomfortable with feeling like I looked "disabled," so I compensated with fast wheeling and jumping curbs. I couldn't bear to be seen being pushed in my chair in public.

Periods of depression began to seep through my heroic façade, as I blamed my paraplegia for my growing unhappiness and loneliness. I had leapt out into public, but was very self-conscious beneath the surface. I was dating, chasing after an idealized love, but expecting rejection. I was awash in unrealistic fantasies of stardom — based reasonably enough on my talents as a musician who started to play at seven and perform at fifteen — but afraid the wheelchair would cost me a spot on the world stage.

In a gradual dawning, rather than a huge epiphany in a moment I could identify, I realized I had been struggling with these feelings *before* I had the convenient scapegoat of my paralysis. My disability had its own issues, and I would need to separate it from what was just about me and the lessons I needed to learn from my life in its own right. I saw that blaming my paraplegia for my unhappiness would mean a life sentence of unhappiness, and that was just unacceptable. This was a key piece of my adjusting to the cold waters of my life.

While the underlying tone of my internal life was a struggle, I was completely independent, enjoying the stimulation of architectural school, having an active social life, and being back on the coffeehouse performance scene, singing and playing guitar. Life was a mix.

My mother and I had remained in our two-story house, where I'd been dragging myself up and down the thinly carpeted steps to my upstairs bedroom. Being six feet two and thin, and with an atrophied, bony butt, this was very unhealthy for my skin. Plus, my denial skills extended to neglecting my weak bladder as I avoided the extra work of using the bathroom, allowing too many catheter slips, exposing my skinny bottom to lots of bacteria. The result? Near chronic pressure sores, which would cost me two extended summer stays in rehab.

In the meantime, I had moved into my own apartment at school (no more stairs to sit on), started using a new external catheter with a double stick band that prevented slips, and become more vigilant about protecting my health. At the inspiration of the owner of a vegetarian restaurant where I'd been performing, I left my meat and sugar diet behind, discovering that broccoli was indeed delicious and that there were far more satisfying and nutritious options than white bread. Besides, I'd already eaten a lifetime's quota of sugar growing up at Karp Drugs.

I had been denying the needs of my disability at my peril. Now I meet my disability on its own terms. Accepting my body and its priorities opens up my options and extends my independence.

In 1979, six years after the fact, I learned that I had not been told the truth about my father. He had, in fact, taken his own life. He had checked into a motel and swallowed a combination of pills that he knew from pharmacy school would accomplish his goal.

It turns out that my charismatic, strong, ex-Navy officer father had lived his life wrestling with deep insecurities, too. I'd always thought that the inner turmoil I felt growing up was a weakness, compared to my father's apparent capacity to work unselfishly, demanding little for himself.

Paralysis only gave me more cause to buy into the image, this impossible way of being. Independence, being a wheelchair showoff, my fight to make my college campus accessible, the music — all of it gave me a false sense that I could indeed hold it together like my dad.

So, learning of my dad's suicide was crushing — but it was liberating. I had a right to my fears and my grief, after all. It would still take years — and support from some good psychotherapists — before I would learn to truly trust what I felt and allow myself to truly grieve and cry when my heart needed to.

I have never blamed myself for my father's choice. My injury was only one factor in the overload of stresses he faced in his life. But to the degree he believed that paralysis would ruin my life, I see him as a victim of the widespread misconception that disability inevitably means a life sentence of loss and strug-gle. His loss motivated me to embrace my disability even more deeply — in all its crazy glory. And I wish he were here to see that he was wrong to doubt I would live the full and active life I have.

My mother never had such doubts. In the emergency room, I heard her say to the doctor that I was not someone to let something like this stop me. In her grief, she still managed to encourage me and keep the household together. Her support carried me through all of this more than I'll ever fully know, but ultimately I had to get out on my own, despite her desire to escape her own loneliness by keeping me around.

After graduating in architecture, and two brief jobs in the profession, I entered a career in graphic design as part of the early wave of computer graph-ics in the early '80s. I fled the suburbs to downtown Detroit where I found the variety and cultural richness of city life much more stimulating. In 1984, when I was twenty-nine, I accepted a job in the San Francisco Bay Area to manage the computer graphics department of a presentation production company. My educational and professional lives affirmed that my disability would not prevent people from recognizing my innate abilities and passion. But I was still alone.

A virgin at eighteen, raised on images in Playboy, I'd been anticipating my first sexual experience in a big way. With my genital sensation and capacity for orgasm reduced, I was afraid I wouldn't be able to satisfy a partner, even though I still felt a very clear sense of my sensuality. Still stuck in my idealized view of perfect love, I was lonely, and insecure on the sexual approach — until my first adult relationship at twenty-one removed any doubt that I could please a partner, that I could be loved. Although it ended painfully, I had made a major transition through sexual doubts, and past the fear that my disability was going to mean lifelong frustration with romance.

Soon after moving to California, when I was twenty-nine, in the heat of the early passionate stage, I married a woman from back home with two sons, before we had the chance to prove our fitness as life partners. I was naïve about the real demands of daily life in relationships. It was an ill-advised quest for an instant family, a way to feel more like an adult — rather than actually growing into one. It was a disaster and ended a year after they came west to join me. Undeniably, part of this experience was a quest to compensate for how I felt compromised by my disability.

Now I know the difference, thanks to my wife, Paula, who I married in September 2003. She didn't see "Gary in a wheelchair" when she met me. She felt our spiritual and sensual resonance, and the potential for what we could achieve together in the space of a real — and realistic — loving relationship.

I was ready for her, having grown through my previous relationships, my work in psychotherapy, and through meditation work I have done since 1987 with a spiritual community called Arica. There I gained tools to increase my ability to observe and understand my life free of judgment. A lifelong process, to be sure.

I learned juggling in 1987 and got connected to a new community of people infused with a creative spirit. It's great exercise, a lot of fun, another outlet for my performance impulses, and a place where I can excel, where my disability is largely transparent.

At the start of this disability journey, I was a youth wanting attention. As I've grown with my disability, my priorities have matured. The point is not to seek attention, but to seek my potential for the good of others. I would not have been capable of making this distinction until I had broken through my unconscious need to compensate for my disability — and begun to transcend the illusions and internal wounds of my youth.

I find it difficult to separate my adjustment to paralysis from my own personal issues, from the karmic map of lessons I believe I'm meant to face in this lifetime. All of these experiences in my romantic, professional, family, and social life have fueled the fire of my personal evolution. Clearly, paraplegia has added fuel to that fire. It is simply integrated into the man I am today — and am still in the process of becoming.

Gary Karp and his wife, Paula Siegel, live in San Rafael, California. He is the author of Life On Wheels: For the Active Wheelchair User, *a comprehensive guidebook for wheelchair users, and an active public speaker. Gary and Paula look forward to making a home for a Labrador Retriever in the near future.*

A Dark Path to God

Vickie Baker
C5-6
Age at SCI: 29
Date of SCI: May 25, 1984
Denver, Colorado

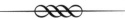

I ran away to join the circus when I was twenty-three. Literally. I was part of a trapeze act, and I loved it! The circus even delivered me my husband, Gary. Every morning I would say to myself, "People aren't supposed to be this happy when they grow up, are they?" Five years later my cherished bubble burst.

During a practice session in our friend Bruce's backyard, I made a split-second mistake in timing, missed connecting with the catcher, and plunged head-first into the trapeze net. On the rebound, from somewhere deep inside, I felt like a coiled spring had snapped. When I came to rest in the net, I could not move.

Help arrived shortly after a frantic 911 call. After an ambulance ride to the hospital with my head immobilized, paramedics rolled me into the ER where X-rays were taken. The neurosurgeon pronounced a verdict of permanent quadriplegia. We didn't believe him. After all, doctors didn't know everything, did they? But deep inside, I worried. What if he was right?

In intensive care, my respiratory doc put me on a ventilator so I could breathe, but it prevented me from talking. The pain from the tube in my throat kept my mind off the doctor's dire statement. In my new motionless, speechless, horizontal hell, I had no way to summon a nurse, so the staff allowed Gary to stay with me round-the-clock to call for help when I needed suctioning. Once my parents — who'd been out of touch for three days — arrived back in town along with two of my aunts, everyone took turns staying with me.

On the nineteenth day, I woke early, excited. It was moving day! I'd "weaned" off the "vent" and looked forward to the roomy therapy gyms, large windows in patients' rooms, and heated pool that Gary described to me. I pictured myself zipping down the halls of Craig Hospital, the rehab center near Denver, until I was back on my feet again. We wanted to get this show on the road!

The first six weeks of rehab were marked by setback after setback. First, my new respiratory doc put me back on the vent. Then, when Gary tried to feed me dinner, the new halo holding my head in place prevented me from swallowing correctly. Instead of sending food down to my stomach, I aspirated it into my lungs. Moments later, my nurse returned with a detestable feeding tube.

They moved me to the Intensive Care Unit of Swedish Hospital, connected to Craig. I'd had a massive gastrointestinal bleed and a high fever, and later learned that I had hepatitis C from the blood transfusions. "You were making such good progress," Gary said, his voice cracking as he turned away.

Finally back in rehab, my therapist got me up in a reclining wheelchair, and I promptly passed out. Gary spent almost every day with me — giving me "tip-backs" every ten minutes to keep me from blacking out. Most quads get over the low blood pressure dizzies after a few weeks. I didn't.

At about eight weeks into rehab, during "chair class" one day, the therapist kept us in the gym instead of doing exercises outside and showed us videos. One of them shattered my plans for the future.

It was about a former patient who demonstrated how she managed various tasks — fixing meals, doing laundry, etc. But I only saw the wheelchair and the curled-up, useless fingers. Her spinal cord injury, at the same level as mine, had occurred over fifteen years earlier, yet she never recovered. I could no longer tap dance around the truth — I would no longer dance at all.

What made me think my fate would be any different? Certainly no one else gave us reason to hope. Doctors and staff pegged me a "C5-6 quad" with an easygoing, casual, "What's-the-big-deal?" attitude, killing my dreams of walking out of there.

Maybe I'd been conning myself all along. Perhaps Gary had too. I had kept my fears to myself on the off chance that I could learn to walk — if I wanted to badly enough. That my fingers would start working — if only I concentrated harder. That the paralysis might completely go away — if I just had enough hope.

Making the ultimate sacrifice, Gary gave up the circus to stay with me. We still lived in our converted 35-foot bus — great for trooping with the circus, but not for pushing a heavy power chair up three steep steps. I left the rehab hospital with the vague notion that I should forget about the past, drink lots of cranberry juice, and accept my lot in life. I did none of the above. Locked up in our own separate worlds of depression, we stopped talking about the future.

That first year, Gary spent all of his time caring for me, which drove us both up the wall and turned our marriage into a nurse-patient relationship, just like a counselor had warned us. We moved into an accessible townhouse the following year. I started using attendants, but our relationship did not improve.

Gary bought a computer, taught himself how to program, and me how to draw holding a pen in my hand brace. While he pored over computer manuals, I began searching out new craft ideas in cutesy gift shops with my aide, Sandy, who delighted in our expeditions as much as I did. When I saw some cute — and very pricey — place mats, I exclaimed, "Craft fairs! The design is so simple, we could stencil something like this ourselves — and I could sell them at craft fairs!" If I could make money at it, at least I wouldn't feel like a total failure.

So we bought fabric, I drew the designs on the computer, and Sandy cut out the stencils. I held the paintbrush in my teeth to paint. I had plenty of stock when craft fair season rolled around in October.

The fairs all bombed.

Gary pointed out that I sold as much as everyone else and that it wasn't my fault so few people showed up. But a small voice taunted, "You're a failure, Little Circus Girl." So much for having faith in myself. A cold chill of despair replaced the light in my eyes. I became focused on my ailments and decided that life wasn't worth living anymore.

The two psychologists we'd seen hadn't helped our crumbling marriage. The doctor I'd visited for my stomach problems, eating disorder, and constant dizziness had no answers. Maybe I just didn't know where to find help. I recalled Sunday mornings in church growing up. The ritual — stand, sit, kneel. Kneel, sit, stand. Repeat mumbo jumbo in unison to a vague, unapproachable God. Could my mother's distant God help me now?

"You never gave Him so much as the time of day," a voice hissed in my ear. "You're worthless, Little Circus Girl. You'd be better off dead. Go ahead, do it," the voice nudged. The dam of apathy burst and dark sinister thoughts sprang to life, twisted ideas swirling through the dark, lonely night.

I learned firsthand that a plastic vacuum cleaner hose melts when taped to an exhaust pipe. I never knew. And how could I have known that starving myself to death would take so long? I figured on three, four weeks tops. Not two months. We would have gotten it that last time, if a friend hadn't called the cops. That won me a free trip to the psychiatric ward and Gary a free trip to jail for ten days for helping me. Bogged down in his own depression, he had planned to die with me. He had already tried once before. Thank God he didn't succeed.

After twelve days of incarceration in a hospital bed, and constant hassles and confusions with the staff amid their efforts to get me to participate in physical therapy, I lay wide awake that night. I had time on my gimpy hands, no control over anything, and there was no way out. A realization swept over me like a tidal wave; I couldn't even kill myself right!

"God ... do you exist? I don't know what to do. I can't die, I don't want to live, and I can't handle everything by myself anymore. I need help!"

I fell into a deep sleep. When my eyes opened, I peered around the room dumbfounded. Daylight. I had slept through the entire night! For the first time since my arrival, I felt well-rested.

Everything that day came off on schedule. I was turned in bed when necessary, positioned correctly, and dressed in time for therapy. It seemed God did exist after all, and He cared about me.

I started noticing that the other patients on the floor, all able-bodied, seemed to have worse problems than I did. Alex had no money. Matt had no place to live. And few had friends on the outside willing to help when they were released. I decided that I wanted do something to help. Six weeks later I left with plans to return to school and got myself accepted into the social work program at a local university.

On the fourth anniversary of my accident, Gary left. I'd seen it coming, but it still hit me like a sledgehammer. In an odd way, it was probably the kindest thing he could have done. It marked a new beginning for both of us. Now I had to stop depending on Gary for everything. And if Gary had worked, I would have lost coverage for my constant respiratory problems, doctor visits, meds, and hospitalizations. No longer prevented from working, chances are he would stop drinking.

Like it or not, the show must go on. Despite the breakup, my disability-related health problems, and my fear of failing school, I survived the first year with passing grades. And I've learned that there is one thing I will always have complete control of — my reactions. If my aide arrives late one morning, or if my ride to the store never materializes, I can choose to be bent out of shape, or I can make the best of the situation and move on. It doesn't mean that I always choose to react in a kindly, caring manner when things don't go my way, but at least I know that no matter what happens, my attitude is my affair.

Despite permanent quadriplegia, a divorce, and a career change (few openings exist for quadriplegic trapeze artists), my present life bears a striking resemblance to the past. When we trooped with the circus, my husband and I built most of our rigging and props. On the road, we needed to improvise if a part broke. After my accident, creative problem solving played an even bigger role in my life, yet it took four years and ten minutes for me to begin. Four years of telling myself that I couldn't do a certain task anymore — like opening and closing my living room curtains — and ten minutes for me to think of a different, economical way to accomplish the goal. Namely, with the cord unscrewed from the wall, I pull it with my teeth.

I hired a new attendant who talked about the Lord a lot, but didn't push it. Mae Lynne mentioned the Lord naturally in our conversations. "My daughter is driving me crazy," she would say, "but every time I talk to the Lord about her, He just tells me to be patient."

Her sincere tone and sense of calmness made it sound like she knew this Lord personally. But she remained perfectly content to keep this mystery to herself — which drove me nuts! She seemed to have a handle on the joy that I had only experienced when leaping out of airplanes or rappelling off cliffs.

She was looking for a new church. Over the next few months, we found the church that I now attend, where I learned that it was possible to have a personal relationship with Jesus Christ, and I asked Him into my heart. Life hasn't been the same since!

My life is now centered on the Lord — not on the trapeze. God has given me a burning desire to write and a passion to live. When I have a bad day, it usually has nothing to do with my disability.

If a cure came along tomorrow, would I sign up for it? I honestly don't know. Without my disability I would be different, and I have no desire to be different. In most ways, I've already been cured.

Vickie Baker, a former trapeze artist turned quadriplegic turned Christian turned freelance writer, has written two books: Surprised by Hope *and* On Wings of Joy. *She and her cat live independently with the help of daily personal assistance in Denver, Colorado. She enjoys reading and tandem-skydiving.*

Surviving Paralysis – Crafting a New Life

Stephen L. Crowder

C4-5

Age at SCI: 38

Date of SCI: August 18, 1995

San Diego, California

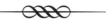

*M*y initiation into the bizarre world of spinal cord injury began innocently enough on the morning of Friday, August 18, 1995. I was living with my girlfriend in a beautiful home in the mountains just outside of Mammoth Lakes, California. For the previous thirteen years I had lived a party lifestyle while bartending at ski resorts and the beach. I was a great athlete and was enjoying a pretty terrific life. I skied, played softball, jet skied, fished — you name it.

My twenty-year high school reunion was scheduled for the following night, so I drove to Los Angeles for a pre-reunion barbecue. The beer was flowing and things got a little rowdy. The next thing I knew I was in the wrong place at the wrong time and swept up in the commotion. Trying to get away from an aggressive drunk, I made an ill-advised dive into the shallow end of the pool, exploding the fourth and fifth cervical vertebrae in my neck.

A friend pulled me out, and carried my limp body to the pool steps trying to reassure me that I would be okay. No, I gently told him. This was it — it was over. I knew my luck had run out. In a way I was right — that was indeed the end of the line for the person I was. But it would prove to be the beginning of a metamorphosis. I would change in more ways than just physically.

My first year as a quad was rough. I'd been living in Mammoth with a large, tight group of friends that would have been there for me every minute, but since it was a rugged mountain town, I had to move. My friends stopped coming around, and nobody called. I felt isolated and alone.

There was so much to deal with that first year out of the hospital. The whole caregiver fiasco was brutal and overwhelming for me. There was so much to figure out — too much. Nothing could have prepared me for the onslaught of problems, issues and paperwork. What did I know about incontinence or insurance dealings? Medical bills lay strewn across my kitchen table.

It was as though I was the first quad ever. Rehab had gotten me from the hospital bed into a wheelchair and strengthened me. They got my health under control while providing me with a basic education about my condition and the care I would require. There was only so much they had time to do, and preparing me for the outside world and all the problems that lay before me was not on the agenda. I was on my own to find the answers I needed. Many of the solutions I needed existed within the minds of quadriplegics and caregivers throughout the country, but there was no way for me to find them and tap into what they knew. I was an island.

I became depressed and unmotivated, but following a memorable talk with one of my attendants, I experienced a life-altering moment of clarity. It was just the old "light a fire under my ass" talk, but she helped me recognize that I had no choice but to fight this war to keep my body healthy. If I gave up, it would just increase the misery, and things would only get worse. I recognized that my life's path would be more difficult than anything I could have imagined, but that's the way it was, and I had better start getting a handle on it before it was too late. If I were to survive, I would have to be more resourceful and more dedicated to the task at hand than ever before. My depression began to lift, replaced by resolve and determination.

I had to turn the page and create a life worth living and enjoying within the boundaries of my disability. I became driven to make the most of my transformed life by discovering new interests and launching different pursuits. And I wanted to pass on the things I would learn by coping and surviving with paralysis, improving quality of life for other people with disabilities. This became my passion.

With my new attitude in place, I came to regard how I responded to my disability and the challenges that came with it as the true measure of myself as a person. I saw that I could explore the potential that was not destroyed in my accident — that still survived deep within me. I knew others who were quadriplegic who had not only survived the transition to quadriplegia, but also lived happy and productive lives. I went to wheelchair chat/information exchange areas on the Internet, to wheelchair sports competitions, concerts, and I saw other quadriplegics doing well. If they could, then so could I!

While I had been a good athlete all my life, my body and athleticism did not define my identity. I had always been pretty intelligent, and it was time to apply myself. I began to develop compensatory strategies, designing adaptive devices and finding ways to make things more accessible. I use voice recorders to keep track of everything, battery-operated letter openers, and a camelback on my wheelchair to have water all the time. I have remote controls for everything. The things I need to be able to grab out of my wheelchair side bags have little loops on them. I designed a strap system with items from a mountaineering shop that allows me to roll myself in bed by putting my hand through a loop and using my biceps. I came up with most of it myself and also recruited friends to brainstorm and do trial and error with me. Someone else would serve as my hands as I described to them what I needed and how to do it.

For years I'd been anxious to get away from the nightclub scene, to reinvent myself. The largest roadblock had always been creating the time. Between work, play and the social life, I always had too much going on. Now I was unable to do all those things — no skiing, no softball, no work. Suddenly I had all kinds of available time, which gave me an ideal opportunity to begin a thorough personal reinvention. I laid down a set of goals — brass rings I call them — and began working on my new life as an advocate and a writer.

As I had done in my teens, I became actively involved in the community as a volunteer. I represent Canine Companions, giving presentations that raise money for the organization to which I feel so indebted. I want to help get more service dogs out there so others can get the boost my dog gives me through the assistance she provides.

All my life I had dreamt of being a sports announcer. My first chance to call a game after my injury was in rehab during a fundraiser quad rugby game between the local team and the nurses and doctors. Still in a halo, I rolled into the gym, got set up and did a few sound checks. "Check one two! Check one two!" My voice felt rich. Then I butchered every name during the introductions, making up cities for all the players. "Starting at right guard, out of Bugtussle, Pennsylvania, number seven, Steve Kaljidjuiski!"

I had announced a lot of baseball games throughout my youth and always enjoyed the feeling I got sitting in the announcer's booth, cradling the microphone in my hands. That night, twenty years later, those same feelings came rushing back to me stronger than ever. I have announced hundreds of events and made all kinds of appearances since, but that first night in the halo was really something special.

After running into an old friend from the University of California at San Diego, the next thing I knew I was auditioning and got hired as the new voice for UCSD baseball and basketball. After that, I started contacting every organization around to get microphone time. I announced all kinds of disability events, youth baseball, you name it. A lot of these events had no announcer. None of the disabled sports had anyone announcing, or else they just threw somebody behind the microphone. I was a natural fit from the beginning. I loved announcing and became the public address voice for the majority of San Diego wheelchair sports and Special Olympics. With my announcing, I could transform any game into an event.

Then I read about a web site where quadriplegics could talk and share information. So I purchased my first computer and, with the help of an old friend, taught myself how to run it using voice-recognition software. It took months of training and practice, configuring my PC, trying different microphones. I found the learning to be both aggravating and exciting, but the ability to speak into a microphone and have my spoken text appear instantly on a screen before my eyes, ready to edit and print, gave me the opportunity to accomplish more than I possibly could with a keyboard.

Finally, I was able to use the Internet and spent two years at the site learning from and advising quads on a variety of issues. Then I reached a point where I felt the site could have been accomplishing more. A lot of these people had nothing else to do and were just on there either bickering or picking someone's post apart word for word.

At this time, a nurse at rehab told me about Dan, a recent quad who desperately needed help. He and his mother were overwhelmed with medical bills, insurance stuff, and all kinds of other red tape. Everyone was stressed, except Dan. His father was in a deep depression and could not face him. He had no personal care system. He didn't even have a blanket that was warm enough or a way to pull it on or off. I met with Dan and his mother for about three hours all the while dictating into my voice recorder. I returned a few days later with a thorough game plan to get him squared away. I had a plan for everything — hiring and training attendants, getting him a wheelchair, getting medications and supplies, straightening out his insurance and billing situation, and much more. I got him all the equipment he needed — even a van by way of donation. I got the family calmed down, his father eventually came around, and my work was over.

I wanted badly to be able to help as many people as possible, but of course there wasn't enough of me to go around. I decided to build a web site that would cut out all the nonsense and best facilitate the sharing of information and support between people with paralysis. I didn't have time to sort through group chat and B.S. for useful information. So I began designing my nonprofit web site, www.SurvivingParalysis.com. Through Dangerwood — the name I call the site — I feel I have fulfilled my goal to help those who are in need to find a way through.

I am accomplishing far more than I ever did before my injury. I persevere. I feel my spirit and determination are stronger than ever, as I continue to handle the serious issues and problems in my life. I have a burning spirit inside of me that is — and always has been — without limit. I've dealt with adversity all my life, so when it comes down to dealing with and accepting my spinal cord injury, what choice do I have? It's not as though I could run away from it — the only way out, is through. Always has been. My survival was my priority and still is, but I have never set any kind of limit on what I — spinal cord injured or otherwise — can accomplish or overcome. I hold on to my dreams and hang on for the ever-bumpy spinal cord injury ride. And, no matter what, I laugh ... and love ... and live.

Stephen Crowder lives in San Diego, California. He is forty-six years old and unmarried. He is an active public speaker, representing organizations such as Canine Companions for Independence and the YMCA, and is the public address voice of local disability events and UCSD baseball. He continues to operate his spinal cord injury support web site, www.SurvivingParalysis.com, and is currently writing a book about his life. He enjoys music and time spent with his dog.

Life Is to Be Lived

Patricia Gordon
L3-4
Age at SCI: 24
Date of SCI: August 10, 1963
Long Island, New York

When I had my accident in 1963, I was twenty-four and had been married for about a year and a half. I received emergency treatment at the local hospital, but I don't remember anything except waking up in bed, attempting to move, and not being able to. I felt very strange. I became alarmed and frightened.

Initially, I was told that my spinal cord was severed. Then, I was told my injury was in the lower lumbar region. I was unable to grasp everything — but I knew it was serious. I became nervous and upset and felt tears rolling down my face even though I was unaware that I was crying. I cried silently. When I was alone, I cried a lot. The future that I had looked forward to — marriage, family, home — seemed gone forever. I was convinced my life was over.

After several weeks, I was transferred to a rehabilitation hospital. Again, I felt that my life was over and was frightened when I saw that I would be living in a large room with many other people. Worst of all was the strange looking, ugly, black bed — a Stryker frame. When I was told that I would remain on it for three months and that I would be flipped over every four hours, I held back tears because my husband, his parents, and mine were also there. I didn't want them to see me crying, and I didn't want them to leave. My husband, Bob, stayed as long as he was allowed. He held my hand and told me he loved me over and over. I cried when they left.

The rehab staff was wonderful — understanding, kind, and patient — but my three months on the Stryker were like an eternity. The next step was being able to sit up. It took longer than I expected. I believed that soon after sitting up, I would get up and walk to the car to go home.

I couldn't accept seeing all the other people — all I ever saw were wheelchairs, walkers, and crutches. I wasn't like them because I would be walking out. When I was measured for braces, I knew I would not be walking without help. I also realized that anytime someone was discharged, they were wheeled out. Yet, being scheduled for a wheelchair class still sounded like a waste of time. I learned all about a wheelchair, its parts, and how to get around safely.

Once I was able to sit up for almost an entire day, I was taken to the Activities of Daily Living area where I learned to do many things I had been doing before. Transferring from my wheelchair unassisted onto the toilet or the bed were difficult new tasks to get used to. I cooperated and tried very hard because I just knew I wouldn't need all this!

I hated using my wheelchair, and I hated seeing so many others using wheelchairs. All I could think of was being discharged and going home. When I was finally able to go home on weekends, I practiced what I had learned in ADL. I didn't like the feeling of being dependent on my husband all the time. However, he never minded helping me and was very happy to have me there. I especially disliked being unable to attend to my personal toileting.

Exhausting exercises and accompanying pain were waiting for me on Monday mornings in physical therapy. The range of motion exercises were especially painful. The therapist, a lovely person, would say, "No pain, no gain." Hearing this didn't help. It hurt!

I enjoyed occupational therapy. I especially liked typing because I had worked as a secretary for two years after graduation from high school. Until I was able to sit, a special device allowed me to type from a stretcher. We also did crafts that eased tension and stress. Doing something "fun" and not painful was great. Day after day after day, the routine was the same.

I worked hard and made friends. Together we shared our common struggles and desires. We became like a family and lifted each other up after our exhaustive exercises. Comparing our painful exercises was serious conversation for us. We preferred the conversation to be about upcoming programs planned by the recreation department and who would be going home and when. Mostly we preferred to laugh and joke. It felt good to laugh. We often avoided conversations about our families to conceal how much we missed them. I no longer felt so alone. I became less moody and much happier. Being with women like myself, I gained back my self-esteem and became comfortable using a wheelchair and seeing others using wheelchairs. We did many things just like ambulatory people. I began to think of the wheels on the chair as my legs.

It disturbed me when I learned of a husband who wasn't able to cope with his wife's accident. I wondered how my marriage would survive. Daily mail from Bob made me realize how lucky I was. Eventually, I was convinced of his sincerity and support. I knew he loved me and wouldn't leave me. Whenever we were together, it wasn't necessary to have lengthy discussions because we were so happy to be together. Our love grew stronger. My fears about my marriage disappeared, and I focused on therapies and being discharged. After eight and a half months, I was ready. Weekends at home had helped me get used to our apartment. Now I needed to get used to being visible.

I thought of myself as "different" and didn't like it. I was certain everyone was staring. People's questions made me uncomfortable. After a while, I could answer politely without going into any details. Eventually, I didn't notice the stares. When curious children asked their parent why the lady was in a "carriage," I would smile and tell them that I used a wheelchair because I was unable to walk. It was difficult to smile when an adult would act like I had a contagious disease and tell their child to get away from me. Thankfully, this didn't happen often.

My adjustment took about two years. Bob refused to let me stay inside and become depressed. My situation would not change — I would not be able to walk. He accepted my mood swings and encouraged me to be happy to be alive. I was fortunate to have such a loving, gentle, and patient husband. He took me shopping, to the theatre, and on car trips during summer vacations. Being in public helped me feel more self-confident.

Bob also refused to let me dwell on any negative thoughts. Still, there were times when I would feel unhappy and "different." I would always miss long walks, riding a bicycle, and dancing. Watching others do these things made me sad and caused my eyes to water. By letting my tears come, I released those negative emotions. I always felt better after crying and talking to Bob.

At home, I had to cope with regular household chores. Changing the linens and handling a heavy blanket or bedspread was challenging. As I approached the washing machine, I felt as though I was staring at an insurmountable obstacle. I wondered how I'd ever do the laundry. By loading the machine in the morning and waiting until the evening when Bob came home and could turn on the dials, we managed. Eventually, I learned to pull myself upright and reach the controls. A long handled "reacher" helped too — and still does.

After about two years, we agreed to look for a new house. We found one that could accommodate my wheelchair. Later, we talked about starting a family. I wasn't at all concerned about taking care of children. I just wanted to be like everyone else on the block. After several miscarriages, we adopted a little boy and named him Glendon. To our surprise, eighteen months later, I became pregnant and gave birth to Laura. It was wonderful feeling normal and being like other families.

Caring for children was not part of ADL. Getting a crib was daunting because I wouldn't be able to reach over the sides to change or dress an infant. Eventually, we found a crib that converted to a youth bed and allowed me easy access.

Chasing toddlers around wasn't the problem that I anticipated. Both Glendon and Laura got used to my limitations and were, to my amazement, understanding. Having a completely fenced in backyard helped because they could go outside, and I didn't have to follow them around. A sandbox, small child's pool, and swing-set kept all of us happy.

Indoors, we read books and played games. Just as I needed to learn to be independent, my children did as well. As they learned to dress themselves, it wasn't easy to watch them struggle. When they cried or fussed, I had to resist the temptation to do it for them — unless it was absolutely necessary. They enjoyed riding on my lap and, later, they learned to stand on the footrest to get anything out of my reach. They understood I just wasn't able to do some things and became self-sufficient. When they were older, Glendon and Laura pushed my wheelchair when we walked to the shopping center.

Sometimes, I have felt foolish remembering the fears about my marriage. Bob has always supported me. Forty-two years later, we are still together.

I have continued typing and have worked at home or done volunteer work. Whenever I volunteer, I feel great helping others and can forget about any problems that I think I have. It's also good to be out. After the fun of OT, I have made various items from craft kits. I took a painting class and find that painting is a great way to forget about myself — even though I'm no Rembrandt. I keep busy and active. Of course, there are still moments when I do miss walking on the beach, feeling sand through my toes, and running or jumping into the water.

Having the love, support, and encouragement of family and friends has been very important. As they accepted me, I accepted myself. Thankfully, during the first year that I was home, my in-laws and other family members stopped by regularly. Friends invited me to lunch; neighbors came for tea. These visits kept me from being alone with my thoughts and getting depressed. More and more, I began to think that I wasn't so different after all. I did just about all the things ambulatory people did. The difference is that I do them while sitting.

There are moments, such as when I need to be carried up the steps of an inaccessible house or when I need to go to the bathroom and it isn't accessible, when sadness or depression occur. Attending a wedding and watching guests dance disturbs me a little less each time. I have come to expect these emotions and believe they are normal. I take one day at a time and am thankful for each one. Most of my days are "up," not "down."

Bob has always told me not to look back. Things cannot be changed, and what has happened, happened. I like his way of thinking. I can no longer go on rides at an amusement park or dance to my favorite music; but I can go to the salon and enjoy getting my hair done just like any other woman, and I enjoy trying new recipes.

I remember my father telling me "you never know unless you try." I don't hesitate to try new things. Besides painting and volunteering, I have cooked gourmet meals, baked, entertained, attended adult education classes, taken piano lessons, learned to knit, and joined a book discussion group. We have traveled by plane to Florida, England, and Scotland. I must always remember to mention that I use a wheelchair in order to get proper accommodations. Going to concerts means sitting in a particular section — and I can never be up front — but I enjoy going.

As a child I was always encouraged to attend church, but my feelings were lukewarm. Now, we attend church weekly and have made wonderful friends. My faith has become stronger from regular church attendance, listening to uplifting music, hearing motivational speakers, reading, and learning to meditate. I am at peace with what happened to me, and I experience less stress and anxiety. I am thankful and happy for each day.

I lead a full life. Today, as a result of changes in society, I do and see more than I could forty years ago. My plan is to continue doing so.

Patricia Gordon lives on Long Island in Westbury, New York. As a busy wife and mother, she has attended adult education classes, volunteered at a geriatric center, with Boy Scouts, 4H, and her church. She has been a member of a Citizens Advisory Committee for the Handicapped, written a column for a monthly periodical, read information onto tapes for use by blind individuals, and has been employed working at home. Recently she began part-time employment at The Long Island Children's Museum.

Beyond the Flagpole

Mitch Tepper
C6-7
Age at SCI: 20
Date of SCI: July 27, 1982
Shelton, Connecticut

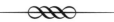

I was baptized into disability on July 27, 1982 while working as a lifeguard. In the moments before I broke my neck, I was twenty years old and in my prime, with sun-bleached hair, a golden tan, and a lean, muscular body. And with an ileostomy bag hidden beneath my shorts.

I wore the bag because a large section of my intestines had been removed earlier in the year. I was diagnosed with Crohn's disease, when it was apparent that I was not growing at the same rate as other twelve-year-old boys. By twenty the disease was no longer manageable with diet and drug therapy. Emergency surgery forced me from college in the spring semester of my junior year, and I was given a temporary ileostomy, which relieved me from pain, cramping, and diarrhea. Since the doctor told me not to let the bag keep me from doing anything I would normally do, I asked for my summer job back as a lifeguard.

Heading out to fix some buoys, I dove over the line that separated the depths. I held a wrench in my left hand, my right over the ostomy bag to prevent it from coming off. This combination caused me to angle too deep, planting my head firmly in the bottom of the lake. I heard a noise from within my head that sounded like air rushing quickly out of a tire. Floating to the surface, I struggled unsuccessfully to lift my head up to take a breath. A fellow lifeguard came to my rescue, asking if I was okay. I said no. I knew I was in trouble.

When I woke up in traction with a C6-7 spinal cord injury, I quickly got the gist of the severity of my condition, and I cried. I have come to believe that acknowledging my condition and letting out my sadness immediately helped me bypass the traps of anger and denial. Eyes wide open, I was able to move on.

I attacked the work of rehab like I had attacked swimming or karate as a teenager. I had self-discipline from sports. I was used to training, so I used those skills and attitudes to do the hard work of training for quadriplegia.

I was deeply concerned about my sexual capabilities from the start. My first sexual question to my doctor was whether I could still have children. I was single at the time and had hardly thought about marriage, let alone being a father. He told me my chances were less than 5 percent.

There was no acknowledgment of my sexual concerns, no discussion about other changes in sexual response I might experience, no referral to someone who might help me with my other sexual questions, and no offer of hope for a sexual future. I was left to work out these issues on my own.

My mother seemed to be the only one who recognized my need for love and affection. From the start, while I was on a ventilator in the hospital, unable to speak, she added the statements "I need a hug" and "I need a kiss" to my communication board so I could ask for it from whoever I wanted — including the nurses. This gave me a vehicle for flirting and the hopes of still being able to express my desires.

My recovery and rehabilitation were riddled with sexually-related experiences, including my reflex erections during bed baths, dressing, positioning, and cathing. Nobody talked about these things — except for one nurse who said "your flagpole is up." The discovery process had started early — in acute care when my family arranged for a girl I was supposed to have a date with to visit me in the hospital, and they set up a romantic lobster dinner. Later in rehab, I dated one of my nurses, having intimate experiences in her apartment just short of intercourse. Also in rehab, I had a sexual encounter with my roommate's sister on a night out on the town that really boosted my sexual confidence.

Then I met a paraplegic guy in rehab who was re-hospitalized for a pressure sore. He reassured me that there was a sexual life for me after all by showing me a picture of his naked girlfriend in a kimono. "This guy is in a chair, and his girlfriend was letting him do this!"

As soon as I could — in the privacy of my bed and still wearing a halo — I began to explore my sexual potential. With minimal arm and no hand function, and an indwelling catheter still in place, I attempted to masturbate. I wanted to know whether I could still ejaculate and whether sexual pleasure was still possible. Having no success, I tried to convince my private duty nurse to help me out. We were about the same age and got along very well. She seemed sympathetic and potentially willing to help, but ultimately was too nervous about her professional boundaries.

As I regained more functional ability, I fought my mother's efforts to keep me home, wanting me to finish school nearby. I was hard on her, ignoring her advice, doing what I wanted, being verbally unkind. Twenty is a key point of independence and separation, and I was already living away most of the time, so the hardest thing was having to be fed and taken care of, being put back into childhood dependency.

I had a strong impulse to rebel and regain that independence, a spirit that I had long held. When I was sixteen or so, in my mother's presence, one of my Crohn's doctors once told me, "Don't let your life revolve around your illness. Incorporate the illness into your life." I had the ammunition I needed to assert my wishes.

I also pushed away the woman I was dating when I broke my neck. She wanted to get married and take care of me. I rejected her like I did my mother because I didn't want to be taken care of like a child.

After finishing my outpatient rehabilitation, I returned to Bryant College in Rhode Island where I had been enrolled as an undergraduate finance major. The college assigned me a suite mate who was on work-study to help with my personal assistance. I was primarily focused on finishing my degree as quickly as possible, but I was still interested in finding a girlfriend.

In the first year following my injury, I took solace in knowing that I could still please a woman. I was not too concerned about my own sexual pleasure — just being able to win over a woman and have sex was my priority. It was a boost to my self- and sexual-esteem once I discovered I could achieve that.

Finding a more serious relationship as a quad — outside the comfortable walls of the rehabilitation hospital and outside the comfortable relationships of ex-girlfriends — was a more risky and painful experience. Some people around me just disappeared. It was painful to be rejected in situations that I knew I would have been accepted in before the accident. I was disappointed, and my response was to become more assertive, making a point to smile at people who were staring at me and to say hello.

My college roommates were actually jealous of the amount of female attention I attracted. What they didn't understand is that the women at school were looking for male friendship that was free of sexual pressure — they assumed I was safe. I was not perceived as a potential sexual partner, but the perennial friend. It proved very difficult to make the transition to being sexual partners.

I felt like I was never going to connect sexually with someone on the level that I wanted — until I met Cheryl in a computer class. My father-in-law always asks us who made the first move. I think she did; she thinks I did. The truth is that there was a real mutual attraction.

I felt totally accepted when I was with her; I did not feel my disability was an issue at all. I had made myself a promise even before I broke my neck that I would marry the first person I dated for six months. I used to date people in high school and early college, two-week relationships that would quickly peter out. I was never into small talk. I would see things weren't going anywhere long term; I got bored, and would move on.

Cheryl and I eased into physical intimacy. We wanted to get to know each other better. She wasn't interested in taking care of me. She looks back on the moment I broke my neck as the event that brought us together.

I used to worry constantly about losing control of my bowels at an inopportune time between the Crohn's and SCI. Then the worst possible scenario happened. I had an accidental bowel movement in bed the first night I stayed over with Cheryl. My heart was pounding, and I broke out in a sweat. I didn't know what to do. I had to wake her, but it turned out that she was cool with this. I was so overwhelmed with this requited love that five months later I proposed. I was afraid if I lost Cheryl I might never find a love like hers again. We were married eighteen months later.

There were concerns from both families because of my disability and our differences in religion — I am an observant Jew, and she is Episcopalian, though she doesn't identify with it anymore. My mother expressed concern about the religion of our children, so I revealed my doubts of being able to father children, having never spoken of them. My mother and Cheryl's parents were also concerned for Cheryl and the burden I would be on her over the long run. Cheryl and I never believed this would be the case.

It has been twenty-one years since my dive into Lake Mohegan in Fairfield, Connecticut, and I have recently celebrated my eighteenth wedding anniversary. Cheryl and I are the parents of a wonderful child, and I've moved from a career in finance to a calling in sexuality education and research focusing on disability. Ours is less traditional than other heterosexual marriages. I clean the dishes, the laundry, and the bathrooms while my wife is the primary breadwinner. Cheryl puts up the shelves, fixes the dryer when it breaks, washes the car, paints, and wallpapers. Our relationship is based on equality, respect, mutual acceptance, trust in each other, realistic expectations, open and honest communication, and flexibility in roles. We believe these are the keys to long term success and happiness — completely apart from any issues of disability.

I was not born into disability secure in my manhood or comfortable breaking out of stereotypic male roles. In fact, notions of what it meant to be a real man were deeply ingrained in me by the time I was twenty. Fortunately, after many years of working on myself, I am relatively free of socially-imposed concepts of male sexuality and masculinity. Yet I still wrestle at times with internalized notions of the male role, as when I prepared to stay home with our son when my wife went back to work. I still feel I'd like to be the primary breadwinner and let her relax. The male image is still at play.

While each man's experience may be different, we still live in a society that attempts to define our identities based on our gender. I've learned that male sexuality goes way beyond who should do the dishes, who should make more money, or the issue of erectile function.

I don't have trouble anymore accepting help. I accept the fact that I have a disability and that it places limitations on me. So I made the transition from crutches to a manual chair, and then to a power chair. It's a process of accepting. I don't need to open every door myself. I actually enjoy being taken care of sometimes — not having to work so hard doing mundane things.

Independence was a very important thing to me twenty-one years ago, but maturation, experience, and learning from others helped me embrace interdependence. I was very involved in the disability community through independent living centers and the National Spinal Cord Injury Association. When I was newly injured, hanging out with people who were twenty years post-injury, I saw how people who needed help could have an identity of independence and still feel good about themselves.

I used to cry every year on July 27, the anniversary date of my injury. There was this underlying loss that I didn't experience every day in my life, but would come up each year. Then one year I forgot about it. I'd reached a point where the quality of my new life trumped what I had lost, and there were no longer any strong emotions tied to that date. I had reached the point of true acceptance.

Mitch Tepper lives in Shelton, Connecticut with his wife, Cheryl, and son Jeremy. He disseminates information and resources on sexuality and disability at www.sexualhealth.com.

When You Come to a Fork In the Road, Take It

Frances Ozur

T12-L1

Age at SCI: 42

Date of SCI: November 6, 2001

Los Angeles, California

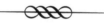

I have always looked at the world through "pragmatic-colored" glasses. Life presents choices, and it is up to the individual to take the path. Left or right, ultimately it isn't going to matter. For me, standing still has never been an option.

Two years ago my future held so much promise. After thirteen years as an electrical engineer, I returned to school to change careers. Eight years, three universities, and two degrees later, in August 2001, I completed my goal and was ready to face the world as a museum curator. Never one to shy away from the dramatic, during the process of negotiating for a full-time position, I collapsed from acute back pain. One clinic, two emergency rooms, one CT scan, five X-rays, one MRI, and one emergency laminectomy later, I woke up to find myself paralyzed from a slipped disc at the T12-L1 level. I had an incomplete injury resulting in cauda equina syndrome (CES). CES is a neurological condition associated with spinal cord injury, including bladder and bowel dysfunction and variable lower extremity motor and sensory loss.

The few months following my operation were a surreal blur of doctors, nurses, and physical, occupational, and recreational therapists all assigned to me during my nine week stay at Rancho Los Amigos National Rehabilitation Center in Downey, California. My social worker helped me contact agencies that provide financial and other types of community support. I had appointments with psychologists who helped me sort out the kinds of changes I was facing. It was the job of all of these people to help me adjust to the physical limitations of a body that no longer functioned as it had for more than forty-two years. With only a thirty percent chance of walking again, it became my job to relearn everything I knew about my life to date. In the before-time, Colin (my life-partner) used to complain that I was "too independent." What I wouldn't give to hear him tell me that one more time.

Today, I am employed full-time as a curatorial assistant at the Skirball Cultural Center in Los Angeles. While I am not ready for any marathons, I am upright and walking — albeit with tons of hardware. I rely on braces and crutches to get around. Talk to anyone who knew me before and they'll tell you I've changed. I had to. Today, I'm more relaxed about life, yet at the same time, I'm much more assertive and self-aware. I no longer play the victim. I found a voice inside — I speak for those who have yet to learn how to. Does all the excess hardware give me courage? I don't think it's that simple. Maybe it was always there and I just never knew how to use it.

It was odd waking up one day to realize that I had become my parents. Thanks to them, I got through this ordeal with my sanity. I remember my father proudly showing me his quintuple bypass surgery scar. He shrugged, "I'm not ever going to ask 'Why me?' because I've had a great life so far. I should be asking 'Why not me?'" I watched this man fight a fatal illness with such dignity, his body giving out as his soul continued fighting passionately. While my no-nonsense father was the realist, my mother taught me to turn the sourest lemons into the sweetest lemonade. It was a blend of these polarities that allowed me to survive rehab by wearing blinders to everything but the immediate task at hand. I blocked out all the things that I was emotionally unequipped to deal with by keeping myself busy. I kept a book with me at all times to read during breaks from classes. I showed up for extra physical therapy sessions. At night, I worked or played on the Internet. I didn't allow myself time to think about what was happening to me.

I enjoyed rehab. I didn't enjoy learning how to go down a staircase in my wheelchair — but I met people from other walks of life that I otherwise never would have. I listened, tried, and soaked in all that I could. I got used to being woken up every morning at 7:30 by my occupational therapist whose job it was to teach me to dress myself. Across the country, my three-year-old niece was learning the same thing. My battle cry echoed hers, "I do it! I do it!" In the beginning, I didn't understand that playing bingo or going to the movies were part of healing. But I soon found out about social interaction sitting in a wheelchair and saw firsthand how people on the outside saw me as someone different.

In the before-time, I blended in. No one ever looked twice as they passed me. Today, people stare and others come up to me and ask, "What happened to you? Did you have polio?" I answer, but it irks me. I still don't visualize myself as different. I joke about my hardware saying, "A girl can never have too many accessories..."

Making a connection with someone who had been through the same thing fifteen years earlier helped me most during rehab. A young woman in my sister's congregation, three thousand miles away, contacted me via email. She mentored me in a way that no therapist could — as she revealed her very personal experiences to me. She taught me that I wasn't alone. She wasn't spouting textbook theory; she was sharing herself. We began our emails laughing over our experiences during occupational therapy classes about paraplegic/quadriplegic sex, and our relationship grew. I had found a supportive sounding board, someone who listened, understood firsthand, and guided me through the changes I was experiencing. Although my mentor's situation was different because her traumatic injury was complete and at a higher level, I learned that all SCIs have basic similarities — bowel and bladder dysfunction, loss of motor skills. She was honest and open, and I will never be able to thank her sufficiently. I know that support groups are available — how lucky I was to find one all my own.

Because of the candor and compassion someone offered me, after I got home, I wanted to serve as a SCI peer mentor. I contacted several individuals at Rancho but there wasn't any such group in place. I contacted a few groups in the state — no one was interested in my help.

I don't think it ever occurred to me that the hospital wasn't the real world, but I learned that on the outside not all floor surfaces are clean and even. In the real world, a nurse doesn't show up if you need help in the middle of the night. That reality didn't set in until my first night at home, and it was very scary. I bought a huge nightstand with drawers and arranged all my supplies so that I could reach them. Since I couldn't jump up in the middle of the night to go to the bathroom, I had to establish a place to keep my catheters, chucks, baby wipes, and even a place to dispose of my waste until I could tend to it in the morning. There are times I really do miss the night nurse.

When I was released from the hospital, I lived alone and had to establish my own local support system. In the beginning, it wasn't easy because my family lives on the East Coast and Colin lived an hour away. It didn't take me long to realize that if I didn't get out of bed, I didn't eat. It took a while before I was confident enough to push a grocery cart around the store. I had to find friends who were really willing to be put to that test of, "If you need anything at all, just call me." Unfortunately the "anything at all" often turned out to be changing soiled sheets. "I do it" aside, it wasn't always a matter of swallowing my pride. I learned to pick which battles are the important ones. Living with SCI makes me focus my energy differently. I have to assess tasks and consider the ramifications on a daily basis. If I choose to do something on my own, will I have the energy to complete the rest of the things I need to do?

I became a planner — a big change for me. Two years after graduation, I still pack my school knapsack every day. I cannot leave the house without meds, catheters, incontinence pads, chucks, a change of clothes, and anything else that I may need. It only took one time of forgetting to pack catheters for work to make them a permanent fixture in my backpack. And, I travel with a charged cell phone because I can't afford to be stuck on the side of a freeway hoping to rely on the kindness of strangers.

I've learned to improvise. During the months before my Social Security Disability payments began, I couldn't afford a gym membership. Colin and I would go to Costco at least once a week because the wide, relatively clean and flat aisles afforded me an ideal place to practice taking steps and later to push a cart and take groceries off the shelves. When I realized that I would need to catheterize myself at work, I brainstormed with my occupational therapist and then invented a new use for the "Itty Bitty Book Light." At home, Colin has rigged up countless devices to make my life easier.

These days, I allow life to happen. I definitely don't take myself so seriously anymore. After leaving a urine puddle in a parking lot a few times, I learned to shrug it off. Even though my mentor had told me this happened to her, I still had to experience it myself. I now wear pads and sleep on an elaborate multi-layered towel/plastic bag system that Colin devised. Because I do have bladder and bowel accidents at work, I've established a routine. If I can, I grab my supplies and head for the restroom. Otherwise, I ask a co-worker to bring me what I need to clean up. It was embarrassing having to show a co-worker where I keep my intimate supplies. But, like it or not, this is my life. I hold my head up and forge ahead. As Winston Churchill said, "When you're going through hell, keep going." Recently when I asked for a privacy door to be installed in one of the museum restrooms that has a shower, human resources agreed that having me clean up at work is more productive than having me leave for the day.

I'm not always upbeat. I do allow myself an occasional bad day. It sucks that this happened. Period. My tap-dancing days are over. There is one person who sees me depressed — the me that I don't care to present to the rest of the world. Colin is the person, for better or for worse, who knows all the secrets. Unfortunately, as my partner, it's his job. Lucky him! I often forget that while this happened to me, his life changed too. This hasn't been the easiest of times for either of us. But history, reliance, and love have held us together. Hopefully, this will be the worst of the "for better or..."

For a long time, I focused on the present — physical therapy and getting through the day-to-day grind of living with SCI. Then, I was able to achieve my dream. I am working in a museum with a staff that is beyond supportive and doesn't care that my legs don't work. I am reclaiming my life. I no longer focus purely on my body. It's not only about me anymore. I am able to give back to my community. I have become an outspoken activist, crusading in the fight to save the rehab facility where this journey began — an incredible way for me to say thank you to all the people who really mattered to me. Earlier this year, I began volunteering with Project Chicken Soup, a Los Angeles based group that prepares and delivers kosher meals for people living with HIV and AIDS.

In December 2002, as my forty-fourth birthday approached, I felt overwhelmingly ambivalent. With everything that had happened, had it been the best year of my life or the absolute worst? I still don't have an answer. But, I'm not dwelling on it. I have things to do, places to go, people to see. I don't know where I will end up, but wherever it is, it's not going to be in the same place I am standing now.

Frances Ozur lives in Los Angeles, California, with her partner, Colin Cole. She recently changed careers, having worked as an electrical engineer since 1980, and is now a curatorial assistant for the Skirball Cultural Center and is self-employed as a graphic designer.

I Will Not Be Denied

Sean Denehy
C5
Age at SCI: 16
Date of SCI: September 8, 2001
Monroe, New Jersey

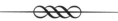

*I*t's the middle of the night, and I am unable to sleep. I lie in my bed trapped inside a lifeless, paralyzed body and do the only thing that I am physically capable of: weeping. In darkness, I search for the answer to one question, "Why did this happen to me?"

On September 8, 2001, I was loving every minute of my first varsity football game. My struggle to make to the team was long, painful, and filled with defeat — but I survived and was reaping the benefits. On the first play of the second half, the ball was kicked and, as the fastest man, I ran to find the ball carrier. I was ready to punish the running back coming full force at me. We collided. A deep bass-like thud reverberated through my body. I didn't feel myself hitting the ground. I knew that my neck was broken.

My father was there; I was terrified. As I was placed in an ambulance, I felt a tingling sensation everywhere in my body. I just cried and made sure that my father gripped my hand tightly.

Three days and two painful surgeries later, the doctors told my family and me that I shattered my fifth cervical vertebra and that the sixth cervical disk was compacted against my spinal cord. They fixed me with two bars, a plate, ten screws, a wire, and a piece of my hipbone. I did not really listen. All I knew was that I couldn't move anything below my neck, and I was scared. The more doctors explained the debilitating effects of my injury, I began to understand the magnitude of it.

Therapy started quickly. But, I wasn't motivated for anything, especially therapy. I still wasn't over the shock. I couldn't stop asking myself why this happened. When I couldn't do what therapists asked, I got aggravated. My aggravation turned to disappointment and then to depression and denial. The realization that I was not able to stand or feed myself was too much for me. Yet, when nurses and well-wishers came to see me, I kept my spirits up for them. When they left, they usually felt better than I did. But when I was alone, I could no longer lie to myself about what had happened.

After a short hospital stay, I was moved to the Kessler Institute of Rehabilitation, where my first day was awful. A C5 sixteen-year-old, ignorant to the world of spinal cord injuries, I was shocked and heartbroken by the people I saw — paras, quads, completes, incompletes. Repeatedly, doctors came in poking and prodding me, performing tests; then, I was left with my family. The one bright spot on this terrible day was when a stranger approached and introduced himself. Initially, I didn't want to have anything to do with him. But, he caught my attention when he told me that he had an injury like mine and had recovered to the point of walking. This was my first experience with how talking with others with injuries could help me.

My feelings became uncontrollable. First, I was unbelievably angry. Then, as the realization of my paralysis set in, I slipped into deep despair and cried. I hit rock bottom. I was empty inside. The vibrant person I used to be had died. The future was a black, dismal cloud, and I was scared to go on. I felt that therapy was going to be pointless if I was just still going to be in a chair. I feared that I was not going to get any better. Yet, through my dark emotions, I told myself that I had to reach deep and rise above this challenge. I told myself that, "I Will Not Be Denied" — not denied of walking, not denied of my self, and not denied of my life.

My family kept me positive by assuring me that they would love me the same — in a chair or not. They and my doctor remained "cautiously optimistic" while making sure that I did not have any false hopes and that my goals were set as high as possible.

The first few weeks of intense therapy were very difficult. My physical and occupational therapists sat me down and answered all of my questions — until I understood what was happening to my body. I was worried that my life was never going to be normal again. I worried that my independence would disappear, about the health of other parts of my body, and that therapy was going to be too hard. Thankfully, they discussed every concern I had and informed me that, while it wasn't going to be a picnic, they would push me to my limits for the best recovery possible. When I was told that I had a chance of walking again, I made up my mind that I would walk out of Kessler on my own. It would be extremely difficult, but not impossible.

During my stay at Kessler, I learned the skills I needed for the outside world, and was able to hang out with other teenagers and make friends with people of all ages who had been injured. Talking to these people and hearing what they were doing for themselves helped me begin to feel more hopeful and motivated. The strength and determination of those who were unable to walk inspired me to reach for my goal of walking again. Talking informally about our everyday lives and even joking about our bowel programs also took a lot of stress off my shoulders. My SCI friends became my "SCI family." We helped each other.

Without realizing it, I shut out most of my feelings and concentrated on getting healthy again. I didn't allow myself to let reality totally sink in, and I kept my mind on therapy. At times, I knew I was shutting my feelings out because I just didn't want to deal with another problem. I would think about something else, watch TV, listen to music, or talk to someone about anything — but my emotions. Other times I was so lost in my denial, I didn't even notice I was shutting everything out. I believe that coping in this way hurt me in the end.

Before my accident, I was self-reliant and self-motivated. If there was ever a problem, I dealt with it myself. Now, I had to rely on others — from getting help off the couch to changing myself. At Kessler, I had kept a lot of my feelings and thoughts to myself. Even though I was offered a psychiatrist, I was not ready to talk about my issues. I just wasn't comfortable expressing my deep inner feelings and discussing issues like going to the bathroom, sex, and death. I did not fully realize how much these issues affected me.

My injury took place three days before the September 11 tragedy. Seeing my father standing next to me, I was able to appreciate the care I was getting, and the love that my family had for me. I thought, "I'm so very lucky." Even though I was still unable to move and faced an uncertain future, the 9/11 victims had it much worse. I continued to think about this whenever I was feeling miserable. Instead of feeling sorry for myself, I was grateful that I was alive with a chance to improve my life

Throughout my football career, I used the motto, "I Will Not Be Denied" to overcome adversity. Now, I used it to help me work harder in therapy and get through tough times. When I was alone, I set tiny goals for myself that I knew I would be able to complete — changing the television channels or doing another set of exercises. I concentrated on the goal and told myself not to fail. When I achieved my goal, I felt great and I moved on to set another goal for myself. When I failed, I knew I had a greater challenge to overcome.

God and my family played essential roles in helping me become physically and mentally healthy. I worried that my body would never get any better, that people would lose respect for me because I was disabled, and that my social life was over. When I was depressed and sad, Mom and Dad would remind me of my progress. My brothers and sister treated me as normal as ever, and my girlfriend was also always there when I needed to talk or have a good laugh. They all gave me the strength and motivation to press forward and remain focused. They were kind and nurturing; yet, they also yelled and scolded when I needed it. They also let me have time to cry and wallow.

During my whole ordeal I turned toward God. I talked to God when I was alone. I had a crucifix hanging above the bar I used to help myself up — He was always there, giving me strength. God helped me cope with why this happened to me. I believe there is a quest He wants me to accomplish. When I look at the world from that viewpoint, it doesn't seem as harsh and unforgiving. With God and my family, I will accomplish what is fated for me to do.

My tiny accomplishments added up. After two months, I was discharged and able to walk to my parents' car by myself. It felt great. But, I did not realize was that my real challenge was just beginning.

At home, I was able to stand and walk for short periods of time. Even though my body was doing great, I was not healed mentally. As an inpatient, it was very easy to shut out my feelings and focus on recuperating. At home, the combination of continuing therapy, tutoring five days a week, and my discovery that my social life was shattered caused a lot of stress. I was getting mad at my family and shutting out my friends who wanted to help.

When the football season started, I lost control of my emotions. I got angry easier and upset faster — and then did not want to deal with anything anymore. I couldn't gather my thoughts about my life or day-to-day issues. I was emotionally unstable. I would go from happy to sad without warning. Sometimes, when I was alone, my emotions were so overwhelming that I would just start to cry.

Right after my injury, I had been told that I would be a coach and very involved with the team during the next season. The reality was that I was too young and inexperienced to be a coach. I was a pseudo-coach/injured player — lost in the shuffle and put in the background to be forgotten. I tried talking to my coach and others to let them know how I felt, but they were unable to understand what I needed.

My emotions were like a roller coaster. My team would score, and I would yell and cheer. Then, I would realize how much I wanted to be out there, and I would fade into background, hanging my head. It was hard to accept my new life while I was still stuck in the old one. I began to realize that I had to move on.

I could either give up on my self and wallow in self-pity, or slowly rebuild myself, stronger than before. When I got depressed, it was damn hard to pick myself up. Talking about my feelings with people close to me — my parents, brothers and sister, my girlfriend — took a lot of pressure and worries off my shoulders. Instead of bottling up my feelings up, I talked about them. Doing this didn't necessarily solve my problems; but it did make me feel better and made it easier to deal with them.

Associating myself with people involved in similar situations allowed me to understand myself and the ordeal I faced. These people showed me that life has its dark times, but there is always someone there to help you. These people — family, peers, whoever — will never cease in helping or loving you either. They help you see how strong you are and offer a shoulder for you to cry on when you feel weak. They make those dark times in your life shorter and less painful. Most importantly, they help you out of these dark times and make sure that you have learned from them. After coming out of this experience, I've truly gained an understanding of how important my family and friends are to me. My family and friends helped me through my injury. I can proudly say that I love my family and am forever grateful for them.

I am thankful that my injury allowed me to learn what is most important — God, family, and the ones I love — and to see that I am strong, mature, and capable. Even though my injury destroyed the life I once had, it started a new one and rested it in my hands. It has shown me the world of SCI, and I will be there to help that world whenever I am needed. Now I talk to people of all different ages who have been injured. I feel fulfilled each time I see them smile and become more hopeful.

I could have given up, but I did not. I will not because "I Will Not Be Denied." My injury has made me who I am and a better person. For that I am proud.

Sean Denehy lives in Monroe, New Jersey. He is currently a student at Villanova University studying in the college of engineering. He comes from a family of six and is very involved with helping others with spinal cord injuries in any way he is able.

Survival of the Fittest

Tiffany Nickel
C5
Age at SCI: 23
Date of SCI: September 1, 1996
Wichita, Kansas

———— ∞∞∞ ————

*D*uring the summer of 1996, I felt on top of the world and believed I could conquer anything. I was twenty-three, had enjoyed some sight seeing in Florida, snow skiing in Utah, and touring in Europe, and was anxious to start my first teaching job.

After eight days of teaching sixth grade science, I was invited to a pool party. Near midnight, I dove into the pool and immediately realized something was wrong. I couldn't move and felt the most excruciating pain in my neck. Friends pulled me above the water, stabilized my neck, and called 911.

At the ER, when the doctor said, "Tiffany, it looks like you've broken your neck," I responded, "That's impossible! Let me see the X-rays." The visual proof was shocking — the fifth cervical vertebrae had a chip of bone detached. After five days in the ICU, I moved to a regular hospital room for seven days to begin my recovery.

Although the doctors explained the reason for my paralysis and the surgery, no one was going to tell me I'd be like this forever. I couldn't move my limbs, brush my teeth, feed myself, go to the bathroom, or sit up — but, it was all temporary. How could it be permanent? My faith had been tested fourteen months earlier by the loss of my mother and brother in a car accident. My life was just beginning to be on track again.

While I awaited my recovery, my anger, and rehab, began. I was angry about my inability to do anything and being at the mercy of the "expert" hospital staff. I hated the insensitivity of the woman who worked with my hands that were all curled up, the tenacious therapists who made me nauseous by forcing me to sit up, the nurse who neglected my right to privacy by emptying my urine bag during the night, and the tasteless food that someone had to feed me. I hated having to rely on everyone for everything!

I hated not knowing how I looked when my friends and family visited. I hated acting emotionally strong because I didn't want anyone thinking this injury had beaten me — pretending was easier than dealing with everyone's sadness and sympathy. My feelings were obvious to my "inner circle" — my dad, stepmom, two best friends, and boyfriend — with my negative talk and outbursts of tears of anger and rage.

I loved the day I got out of that hospital. But, why was I going to another hospital? Why wouldn't anyone tell me when this spinal cord injury would heal and I would walk again?

At the rehab hospital, I told everyone I had to be out in a week to work at the state fair, and I told my friend I could still be in her wedding in two weeks. I would be fine. Almost everyone was verbally optimistic about my recovery — but, who knew what they were really thinking? Cards, calls, and visits all included phrases like, "You'll beat this" or "You're so strong." I told myself that I'd be "normal" again. "I've always helped others — Girl Scouts, 4-H, Special Olympics, The Association of Retarded Citizens, or teaching. No one needs to help me!"

Awaiting normalcy, I was made to continue the obnoxious and rigorous rehab work — sitting up and trying to balance, stretching, rolling from side to side, transferring, moving objects from one bowl to another with my fingers, wheeling around the gym, and looking at catalogs of devices that I didn't want. It all seemed so meaningless. I avoided believing annoying staff members —

who had the audacity to tell me this paralysis was permanent — because their experience seemed limited. Except for a young man and me, the other patients were all seniors recovering from strokes, hip replacements, or the complications of diabetes.

The physiatrist discussed physical, occupational, and recreational therapy, medicine, bladder and bowel management, spinal cord education ... blah, blah, blah. What was quadriplegia? Why did he keep calling me quadriplegic? I still wanted proof! Once I saw the titanium in my neck and the bruise on my spinal cord, reality began to set in, and I cried more often — but only around my "inner circle." Fearing I would break down and cry and show my weaknesses, I refused to see other visitors.

I hated getting up each day, going out of my room, or seeing the sunshine — my depression had begun. I denied it. But, my inner circle knew it, forced me out of bed by scheduling my therapy sessions in the morning, and urged me to talk with a counselor. I refused counseling because being "strong," I never felt I needed "help" — and my past experiences with counselors hadn't seemed worthwhile. Why would they be worthwhile now?

At this point, the last thing I wanted to deal with was wheelchair users. But, this was impossible. My case manager was paraplegic, and people in wheelchairs kept visiting to tell me how great their lives had become. I believed that therapists were taught to integrate positive wheelchair users into the new patient's life — whether I liked it or not. Did they think I cared? I wasn't going to be paralyzed forever.

During the next three months, I began to learn to wheel, transfer, write, feed myself, brush my teeth and hair, bathe, semi-dress myself, and apply make-up. I chose a wheelchair and became familiar with Velcro and the necessary activities of daily living equipment and supplies I might need. When I toured the dream home that my dad had built a few years earlier to assess the modifications — widening doors, building ramps, and reconfiguring bathrooms — I would need, I was overwhelmed by the cost and time required and felt guilty.

I had become attached to the nursing staff. They knew my personal needs and treated them as normal. When discussing my bladder and bowel care, they taught me to find some humor in it. They treated me as me — not a paralyzed patient whose body was out of control — and became my extended family.

My room was covered, wall-to-wall, with cards and artwork from the sixth graders I only knew for eight days. On a day pass, when I visited my class, my students' compassion and acceptance motivated me to regain some sense of normalcy — by hanging out with friends and family, educating myself about SCI, and preparing to return to teaching.

When discharge day arrived, I was delighted and terrified — about life without the security of twenty-four hour care, level entrances, smooth floors, accessible bathrooms, and people who understood and accepted me. On the drive home, I was filled with anxieties about surviving at Dad's house, becoming my new self, and what others would think about me in a wheelchair.

At home, I began to test myself and became angry and frustrated when I couldn't move my wheelchair on carpeting, reach sinks, open doors, or prepare food — and when people couldn't read my mind and rescue me. No one had told me how to become less dependent on my family for everything. Something had to happen. I couldn't continue living that angry.

Somehow, my lifelong independence and stubbornness and the thoughts of my students awaiting my return helped me survive. I developed a "Survival of the Fittest" mentality because nobody was around — my inner circle had to live their lives and return to work. Slowly, I mastered transfers, because I got tired of waiting for others, and pulling myself up in bed, because I felt guilty waking people up at all hours. I had to rely on myself.

Hearing that there were people my age, including women, and an experienced staff and fine facilities at Craig Hospital in Denver, I was easily convinced to fly there myself for five weeks of intensive rehab to improve my level of independence and take driving lessons. I was ready to live productively as a disabled woman.

At Craig, I was surrounded by people my age in an environment that encouraged me to improve my physical independence and heal emotionally. It was like a club for the young and paralyzed — women and men from many backgrounds as well as staff members who were wheelchair users. I was excited to meet people like me, realized I wasn't alone, and discovered that my scenario could've been worse. I didn't want to miss any opportunity to meet someone or learn from a peer. Everyone had a story to share and their own approach to mastering paralysis. Through trial and error, we tackled laundry, catheter bag connections, and shopping. Taking it all in, I even found it hard to sleep!

I was inspired by a woman, in for re-evaluation, who was able to live independently, return to college, connect with disability Internet chat rooms, and continue dating. Another young, recently-married, quadriplegic who had just started her obstetrics and gynecology practice, was also inspiring. Her focus was on returning to her profession, but she frequently cried, fearing that her goal might not be attainable. Like me, she was surrounded by family, but was comforted by her disabled peers. She was empowered by leading a support group on the reproductive cycle and SCI in women.

I constantly pushed myself to improve. I was proud and greatly relieved to master dressing, bowel/bladder management, transfers, etc. and, most importantly, driving. I could decrease my reliance on my inner circle, give them their lives back, and gain control of my life. A "ton of bricks" was lifted off my shoulders.

The Craig staff was outstanding — experienced, honest, and down to earth. They empowered me by calling me "Superquad," reassuring me about my progress, speaking positively, involving me in groups with peers for exercise, support, and recreation, and sharing stories about others' successes and capabilities. They never missed an opportunity to educate me or let me educate a new patient by demonstrating a certain skill. The fact that they trusted me enough to teach others was a huge motivator and self-esteem booster — I felt worthwhile and capable. I continue to enjoy visiting Craig.

All my encounters with SCI survivors, individuals working with the SCI community, and every child in my life have helped the last seven years come and go. They encouraged me to meet the challenges and opened my eyes to my successes — even with quadriplegia. I've accepted my paralysis and always remind myself of the positive and loving words of my family and friends. I've also accepted that everything takes longer and requires more patience and determination. Yet, there isn't a day that passes that I don't hope for a cure.

My parents had taught me the importance of determination, perseverance, and goal-setting. By focusing on my goals to get back to teaching and be as independent as possible, I made it off the roller coaster of denial, anger, depression, and guilt — several times.

When the challenges of everyday life cause moments of anger, self-pity, and frustration, I stop and remind myself that there are worse case scenarios. I could be unable to communicate or move my arms, or not be surrounded by loved ones.

I still get angry — when someone parks on the lines for a wheelchair ramp and blocks me in or out of my van, or when something limits me from living my life as normally as I can. But I've learned to breathe deeply and complain politely, and remember that the squeaky wheel gets the grease. I'm grateful to anyone who offers help.

I educate everyone I can by sharing my story honestly and explaining that nothing is attainable without hard work, determination, and some failures. I also seek out others who have been injured and participate in local support networks — listening and learning from others within the disability culture. Now, I am a special education teacher and a role model to my students, focusing on "if I can, you can."

I live by myself, own my home, and hire attendants (five mornings and three evenings each week) to make life easier. Besides teaching, I keep busy volunteering — as executive director of the Kansas Disability Coalition, secretary of Wheelchair Sports, Inc. in Wichita, with my college alumni, and in my church.

I continue to surround myself with amazing people and thank them all the time for their support. My inner circle, who accepted my daily struggles and my emotional recovery roller coaster, continue to be a source of strength, inspiration, and encouragement. They have helped me by listening when I ranted and raved, laughing with me, and giving me the power to laugh. They never left my side and always treated me as normal Tiffany, not as quadriplegic Tiffany.

Tiffany Nickel lives and works as a special education teacher in Wichita, Kansas. She enjoys family and friends and serving as a board member of Wheelchair Sports, Inc. and as the executive director of Kansas Disability Coalition, Inc.

I Don't Want to Fail

Nicolas W. Libassi

L1

Age at SCI: 26

Date of SCI: November 16, 1996

Clifton, New Jersey

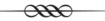

When I was 22, I decided to try skydiving. Parachutes and free falling always fascinated me. As a boy, I can remember using a plastic bag and thread to make a parachute for my G.I. Joe doll. I would throw him off the roof and watch him fly.

On November 16, 1996, I was involved in a mid-air collision and plummeted 15,000 feet. I never lost consciousness. At the hospital, X-rays revealed an L1 burst fracture resulting in paraplegia.

Before the accident, I had a life plan — marriage, children, a home of my own, and a good paying job. Lying on my hospital bed, I thought that none of my dreams were going to come true. How was I going to meet a woman able to accept my condition? How could I have children? Who was going to hire me?

My depression was worse than the actual injury. I did not want to get out of bed or eat. I had nothing to look forward to, and no hope for the future. I could not snap out of it. I went to rehab every day and felt like I was just going through the motions. When I met others who were paralyzed and they talked about life in a wheelchair, I did not want to hear about it. I felt that they were bragging about how they made it through.

Although I did not want to be there, rehabilitation was a great tool to keep my mind off of negative thoughts. As I did my various exercises, I focused on getting back as much function as possible and maintaining whatever function was left. My therapists kept me thinking positively. They pushed me to be independent in everything that I did and taught me how to transfer from a couch or a car and how to take a shower by myself. They also spoke about what I could expect when I was released and assured me that as time passed I would be happy. This was essential for my motivation.

While I was an inpatient, I was assigned a psychiatrist just like every other patient. I was not ready to speak to her and have her analyze me, but I had no choice. The sessions were dreadful. Pretending that I was not at all depressed, I would just tell her what I thought she wanted to hear and hoped that she would discharge me. She asked personal questions that I felt had absolutely nothing to do with why I was there — about my friends, my family, and my girlfriend. Whenever we met, my resentment toward her grew. I felt that she was just doing her job and did not really want to get to know me. I was not ready to speak to a stranger about my deepest emotions.

I believed my inside emotions were all that I had left. I had lost a key part of me physical identity, and I was scared to give up my feelings — my emotional identity. I worried that she would draw all of this information out of me and that it was going to make me weak. I had strength and control over what I divulged to her. This was important to me because I had nurses helping me go to the bathroom, get dressed and showered — almost every aspect of my daily life. I felt I had no dignity and no control over this. By holding on to my emotions, I felt in control of something. And, I had my physical recovery to worry about.

Once I was home, my depression became more intense, and I began to think of different ways to end my pain. Suicide was constantly on my mind. With the amount of time that I had on my hands, I imagined many ways to kill myself — roll into moving traffic, throw myself off a building, and even drive my car crazy to get the cops to chase me and then pull out a fake gun so they would shoot me. I was in such a dark place. Now, I feel ashamed that I actually had such thoughts. Before I was injured, I had wondered how life could get so bad that anyone would commit suicide — now I understood. I never had so much time on my hands. Lying in bed for hours at a time, I had too much time to think about negative things — I was never going to get a job, get married, or have children. I thought that my life was going to be horrible.

With the help of an incredible family, I started to see the light at the end of the tunnel. My parents and siblings were with me all of the time. They kept telling me how everything was going to be all right and how proud they were of me for being so strong. Speaking words of encouragement to the point that it made me nauseous, and not allowing me to become secluded, they showed as much courage as they thought that I had. I felt that I had to get through this so they could get on with their lives — and know that I would have a good life.

This is the first time that I have expressed my feelings about suicide. I am not proud of having had such feelings, but I know it is an important topic because many newly-injured people think about it. I am so thankful that I am still alive and can go on. I have a lot of things going for me. At one point, I decided to make a list of things that I had to be grateful for. When I was finished, I realized there was no reason to feel so down about my future.

I prayed to God to watch over me, give me strength, and guide me to all the things I so desperately wanted. I spoke to Him often and this really helped me. I felt like I was giving my worries away. This was the start of my emotional recovery. Little by little, I started to do more — going to the mall, out to dinner, and just being in public. Getting out made it easier and easier to be with people.

At about that time, the New Jersey legislature was considering a new bill to raise money by allocating one dollar from every motor vehicle violation fine to research to find a cure for paralysis. It may seem hard to believe but I wrote thousands of letters to friends and family members urging them to write to their local elected officials to support this bill. I received letters from several state legislators stating that their offices were inundated with letters that mentioned my name. I was proud to be invited to the ceremony when Governor Christine Todd Wittman signed the Spinal Cord Research Act.

A few years later, because I was starting to cope with my injury and wanted to speak to someone other than my family members, I went to a new therapist. I was ready to address some of the things that were making me depressed. This time it was awesome! She was so nice the first few times that we met, and we talked about everything but my injury. She took quality time to get to understand who I was. Her questions were non-probing, and we just had good conversations. Once we got comfortable with one another (I also learned a great deal about her and her family), she was able to help me figure out my depression by helping me explore my feelings.

A major part of my depressions was that I secluded myself from my friends after my accident. I did not want to go out with them or even speak to them on the telephone. She helped me understand that I was still the same person and that I needed to speak to each of my friends individually and explain my feelings. Although it was awkward, I had to tell them about how I managed my bowels and bladder and about my major fear — that I would be put into a situation that was uncomfortable and embarrassing. By sharing this information, my friends could understand what I had been through. By explaining my needs, they could make sure that I was not going to be embarrassed. These conversations also helped my friends to see that I was no different mentally.

It was so exciting to have my friends back. I started to do more and get out of the house more — a tremendous part of my emotional healing. My therapist also helped me see that I could do anything that I wanted to do. She stressed that while I might need a different approach now, if I put my mind and heart into it, I could achieve my goals. She became a personal friend. Now, I know that I had to want to express my feelings in order for psychotherapy to work.

One year after my injury, I started to think about working again. Before my accident, I was a workaholic and never was able to sit still. In any spare time, I was active playing basketball, baseball, softball, football — and skydiving. I did not tolerate being unproductive. My only work experience was as a carpenter. I had owned my own company since I was nineteen. When I thought about what I wanted to do, I realized that all of the construction jobs that I had gotten were due to my ability to sell my services and skills.

I decided to look for a sales position. I went on some interviews with confidence in my ability and forgot about my disability. My confidence probably came from the fear of rejection. Before long, my fear subsided and I was more confident with who I was. I got several offers. I decided on one, did very well there, and gained experience in a professional setting.

Then, with more knowledge and experience, I wanted to find a better paying job with better prospects. Several interviews later, I was offered a position with a fine company. I soon became the top producer and gained unbelievable respect from my peers. I worked for a couple of years for that organization, but then I felt I was not going to be able to climb the corporate ladder. I was given an incredible opportunity to work as a sales representative for one of the largest companies in the world. I have been successful in my professional career because I display all the positives that I bring to the table — including my ability to be honest and form lasting relationships. And, I treat people as I want to be treated. Most of all, I am sincere and passionate about succeeding.

I have dated a few women through the years. None has seemed just right for marriage because I am very picky and look for certain things — different things than before November 1996. The biggest difference is that I now try to see a woman as a complete person rather than just a sexy body and a cute face. I want someone who cares about me and shares my beliefs. She must want to better herself without changing who she really is, she must love me for the person that I am and not because of my disability, and she has to have a strong sense of family. Because I have met many men with paralysis who have fathered children, I am confident that when I find the woman of my dreams, I will have the same opportunity. It is not easy to find the right person to spend your life with. But, in my opinion, that has nothing to do with using a wheelchair.

Today, almost seven years since my accident, I am still striving to achieve my goals. Nothing comes easily, every day has its challenges. The simple fact is that when something needs to be done, I have to do it. The more I do, the more positive my attitude becomes and the more I get done. Time spent thinking about all the things that I cannot do takes away valuable time from achieving and maintaining happiness.

I have stayed positive because I do not want to deny myself all of the things I dream about. I know that I am no different from an able-bodied person. There are things that they can't do either. I can honestly say that I very seldom get down because I know how lucky I am to be here today.

My life isn't perfect. But I believe that I have found myself and am comfortable with who I am.

Nick LiBassi lives in Northern New Jersey. He is a product consultant for a large company and is working toward his business degree. He has spoken to many groups on what it is like to live with a disability.

In Competition with Myself

Randy Snow
T12
Age at SCI: 16
Date of SCI: July 28, 1975
Terrell, Texas

⚬⚬⚬

I came from a large family. My parents were well-to-do, upper mid-dle-class entrepreneurs, with master's and law degrees. We had a lake house and loved to water ski, had a small private airplane, loads of time for recreation, and of course, very high expectations. These attributes, assets, and burdens formed my sixteen-year-old, able-bodied makeup.

I loved sports, from pony league baseball to high school football and basketball. I participated in every kind of competition I could find. I was a ranked tennis player and had high hopes of landing a scholarship at my hero school, the University of Texas. Sports were my foundation, my love. Me.

In the afternoon of July 28, 1975, using a hydraulic front-end loader at a summer job, I attempted to lift a single 1000-pound bale of hay and place it on a flat bed trailer. As I began to ease the hydraulics back, the bale dislodged and fell on top of me, pinning me against the tractor. Four of my ribs were broken and my right lung was punctured. My humerus had a compound fracture and my twelfth thoracic vertebra was crushed. I was permanently paralyzed from the belly button down.

Transferring to Craig Hospital near Denver, the term "rehabilitation" entered my quickly expanding medical vocabulary, along with several other unappealing terms like "atrophy," "catheter," and "muscle return."

Everything that had defined my life, that I considered enjoyable and rewarding was gone. Walking through the woods, hunting and fishing, a cramp in my hamstring, the feeling of new blue jeans on the first day of school, water skiing, running to the net to shake my opponent's hand — my freedom, my future, my plan — all of it was gone. The thought, "This can't be happening" dominated my thinking. On the outside, I presented the mask of, "I will handle this." Inside, I had no idea how.

Paralysis was very bizarre. I had to start over and learn to do things as an infant might. I was naked most of the time, peeing and pooping on myself, unsure and dependent on people for just about everything. Privacy was nonexistent. Everything from my personal hygiene to social and spiritual needs were an open book to each staff, patient, and family member in rehab.

As a self-assured athlete who understood his body, now my new vessel continuously baffled me. I could comprehend the medical fact that part of me was paralyzed but it didn't help with the overriding feeling that, in a way, I was being abandoned. I felt like two people.

In the acute hospital, I had run the show, so I imagined I could do the same in rehab. My therapist, Beverly, arrived in my room the first morning, saying, "Good morning, Randy. Let's get going to the gym." But King Randy had decided to spend the first few days in his room, so I said, "I think I'll stay here until tomorrow." Bev had another vision. Ignoring my protests, she unceremoniously unplugged my hospital bed, pushed it down the hall, into the gym, and left me there in the corner. I had no choice but to lie there, scared to death, taking in the personal efforts of the other patients at work.

I arrived at rehab with the belief that there could be no dignity in a life from a wheelchair. I expected the wheelchair world to be filled with pity and sympathy and heroic effort — and I didn't want any part of it. Before my injury I was an athlete, a competitor, used to laying it on the line. My life was one of sacrifice and preparation, of high-level performance. Being so aware of my physical past made the task of accepting paralysis seem almost impossible. I was having an extremely hard time, regularly escaping into fantasies about what I used to be able to do.

The kindly hand of time eventually softened my non-compliant attitude because I guess I got tired of holding on. It just became more painful to stay the same than it did to change. As an athlete might, I began to take on smaller goals, seek interim achievements, focusing on the immediate challenges. Little victories like dressing myself or independently transferring out of my bed distracted me from obsessing about the ultimate goal — going home. And, of course, walking.

Rehab was a matter of doing things one minute at a time. Getting dressed on my own for the first time was a huge turning point. Putting pants on paralyzed legs was like putting on wet socks times a hundred. All of us asked our families to bring the easiest clothes to put on that we could think of. My entire wardrobe consisted of cotton sweats and big T-shirts.

I cannot begin to express how important my rehab team was at Craig. There was an ambitious commitment to a common goal. Initially I considered them the enemy. They quickly became my soldiers. To this day I keep in touch with several of my therapists.

The most invaluable influence in my reformation was the faith and support of my family and true friends. They say that fear cannot exist where there is faith. They had faith in me, which gave me strength. I couldn't imagine telling my family that it was too hard or that I wouldn't make the effort. Having them to talk to and to share the pain with had a huge impact during the early stages. To let them down would be to let myself down.

Sometimes love has to work from the other direction. After discharge, one by one my mother reduced the list of tasks she did for me. Rather than enabling me into dependence, she started staying out of the way. It was difficult to swallow, but I learned that the family members who seem to be the hardest on us, are sometimes the ones who love us the most.

For some strange reason, I thought if I could just get out of rehab and go home, everything would resolve itself. Everyone in Terrell, Texas, anticipated my return yet no one, including myself, had any idea what to do once

I got there. With more innocence than pity, most embraced me. But even though I knew I was the same person, several of my high school acquaintances were not able to face what turned out to be their own hang-ups. My lineup of friends began to shift.

My pseudo-acceptance lingered for about three years. I avoided other people in wheelchairs, crossing the street if they approached me. Then someone suggested wheelchair sports. Are you kidding me?! But in a weak moment I attended a wheelchair basketball exhibition. I sat on the sideline hoping they wouldn't come over and speak to me, but naturally one of the players zipped up and asked if I wanted to join in. Offering a perfunctory, "No thanks," what I really thought was, "Man, I was a real athlete — I don't play in a wheelchair."

Through the risk taking, development of thick skin, and the priceless quantities of time that were my path to acceptance, I ultimately arrived at the rediscovery of the joy of competition. Once I allowed wheelchair sports in, I pursued them with voracious passion, and felt immense relief and a sense of reward. Hearing people once again telling me that they were impressed with something I did fueled a fire and generated energy that motivates me to this day. I wanted to be accepted. It was my psychological background — a selfish kid that worried about what other people thought. I did not want other people to think I was soft. Competition was my self-esteem mechanism.

Wheelchair sports is not easy, which is exactly why it has been so pivotal for me. Dreaming, setting goals, pushing my limits — sports acts as a prism for me, separating out my fears, rigid beliefs, insecurities, and ego. Sports allows me to see all these parts of me, helps me understand who I am and what I can do. After training 100 miles a week for a year and racing in front of 80,000 people, interviewing for a job seemed simple. Sports reminds me that life is about tests, and if we don't get it the first time, we recycle. We get back up.

Wheelchair athletics gave me influence, a way to affect cultural attitudes. When someone sees me playing tennis and thinks, "Wow. I didn't know a disabled person could do that," then maybe they won't jump to the usual negative stereotype but reconsider what's really possible with a disability. And through my accomplishments, I've been asked to support advocacy and legislation. I'm always pleased to be asked to show up for advocacy events, like some I experienced with disability pioneer Justin Dart and for the activist group, ADAPT. I'll always do what I can if my sports image can help improve society.

Giving up is easy — deciding not to cross that uncomfortable boundary and try something scary. And it gets easier and easier each time you do it. Sports taught me to reverse that habit. There's a huge payoff when you keep up the effort, when you face what is daunting, and don't give up.

The key to longevity with a disability is to augment my circulation. Since half of my muscles are not being used, and are below my heart, exercise enhances the movement of blood back to my heart. Staying active keeps my weight at a minimum, which helps digestion, respiration, muscular development, transfers, and all aspects of life. I can push a grocery cart today thanks to pushing a racing chair through airports around the world. I can transfer into an oddly-positioned bathtub thanks to doing transfers up into my basketball chair after a collision on the court. Preparation for marathons was the same as getting in shape before a recent ten-hour back surgery. What I've done for sport has spilled over into all of the key areas of my life.

Competition has contributed to the social aspects of my life. I traveled overseas with U.S. teams, and have encountered the many beautiful and different people of the world. Being around other ambitious and goal-oriented disabled folk showed me the shortcuts to function and adaptation — an empirical "Spinal Cord Injury Manual." When I was still recently-injured, it was invaluable to observe a seasoned wheeler deal with an inaccessible restroom in Tel Aviv or do a transfer into a kayak.

Sports helped me develop a healthy body image, to regain my assertiveness and accept my new self. A half-marathon challenges my ability in many ways, but what I gain most from taking the risk is self-esteem. Sports filled the gaps and taught me to problem solve and use resources efficiently. There is no space left for a self-image of being weak.

Sports brought me to spirituality, which helps me cope with myself and with others, to be a vehicle for change, to find a sense of purpose. Perhaps the medals they've given me transform once I take them home and become the ones I try to place inside other people to help them reach their potential. Winning a gold medal has pushed open a window to my soul where every emotion I've ever felt is kept. It begged the question of what is really important: that I win this match or that I value the experience? Sports taught me to think less *about* myself — and more *of* myself. Humility is having an ego that is just the right size.

I suppose my injury can be seen as sort of an athletic competition. I was deeply into the game of life when I experienced a drastic change. I was faced with a decision — what was I going to do? The philosophy of any great athlete is that, when you initially face defeat, you accept it — and then you take action. This is the process I have constantly used, and I'm grateful for this little life tool that gets me to the other side where I truly learn about myself. My job, as usual, is to just stick around long enough for the miracle.

Randy Snow lives in Terrell, Texas. While he is single, his four sisters and their children make "Uncle Randy" their top choice for babysitter. He is an inspirational speaker, author, and Olympic and Paralympic medallist. In what little spare time he has, he spends it fishing, exercising, and reading.

The End of Denial

Don Bondi
C5
Age at SCI: 18
Date of SCI: May 10, 1969
Aliso Viejo, California

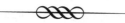

I thought I was pretty smart when I was eighteen. I never drove when I was drinking, and I never rode with anyone who was drinking. Except once.

After a party in Trabuco canyon, I caught a ride with my friend Del. We'd waited a couple of hours to sober up, but still Del lost control of his '58 MG and crashed through a guardrail. He landed on the rocks, and I landed in the sand on the dry creek bed. When I came to I tried to get up, but nothing moved. Strangely, there wasn't any pain. I could hear Del's heavy, labored breathing, and I tried to talk to him. I wanted to help him but couldn't, feeling guilty that I was in no pain but could do nothing.

I don't know how much time passed without any response from him until I realized he had stopped breathing. I can't remember what I felt at that moment. My brain just shut down. The next words I heard were from the rescuers, finally arriving, saying, "this one's still alive."

It was 1969, before the time when they would put a collar on you and tape your head to stabilize it — precautions that are standard now. They just thought I was drunk, even though I told them I thought I had a spinal injury. In the emergency room, they still treated me like I wasn't seriously injured, lifting me up to get my leather jacket off and undressing me. I was barely conscious and in shock, so I barely knew what was happening. When the doctor arrived, he realized what was wrong, and at last they started handling me with care.

My parents were at the emergency room when I got there, and they weren't handling it very well. After the initial shock and not knowing if I would live, the emotions started pouring out. My mom was crying and emotionally out of control, thinking it was all her fault. She had bought me a six-pack of beer that day. My stepfather was trying to comfort her, not knowing what to do. Dad was holding up in front of me, but I could see he was holding back the tears. My stepmother, Harriet, was crying and holding on to Dad.

My eleven-year-old sister, Julie, was kept in the dark because they felt she was too young to understand. A week or so later I asked for her. She was afraid so I tried to reassure her that I was all right. We spoke only briefly, but I told her I loved her. We were always close but years later she told me that this was the first time I had said this to her.

With my family in such an emotional state, I felt that I had to be strong for them, so I stuffed my fears, anger, and uncertainty deep down inside me. This was the beginning of my own denial.

I spent three months in the hospital after my C3-4-5 spinal fusion, then was transferred to Rancho Los Amigos to begin rehabilitation. Because I was never in pain I told myself that I would recover. My dad and Harriet shared my denial, always talking about me getting better. One day during rounds my physical therapist said, "You'll probably never walk again." She could tell from the look on my face that I had never been told that — much as I suspected it was true. I saw the disappointment and pain in Dad and Harriet's eyes when they heard the news. It suddenly slammed me in the face; I had been so deeply in denial that I didn't think I was in denial at all.

I was never the same easygoing guy after that. Gradually I became angry, treating the aides and nurses badly, being very demanding and verbally abusive. Unconsciously I resented them for doing for me what I could no longer do for myself. One night the nurses told me to stop yelling or they would remove me from the room. I didn't, so they did. After this I got to thinking that I could fight this all the way — or I could treat people the way I want to be treated. I made a choice to turn my anger into motivation and work hard.

Aside from the great rehab at Rancho, the best thing that happened to me there was David and Gail, friends of my girlfriend. I met them a few days after my arrival. They took me out on weekend passes and helped me re-acclimate into the real world. I felt uncomfortable with everybody looking at me wherever I went, but they wouldn't let that stop me. They dragged me out anyway, asking, "How many people did *you* see in a wheelchair before your accident?" None I could remember. They wouldn't let me feel pity for myself but were sympathetic when I needed it. They did something that not even my family could do — they treated me like a person. Just another friend, not "special." I didn't have to be the strong one around them.

The five other quads and paras in my room were important to my success in rehab, my realization that there was going to be life after my injury. We would kid each other and tell big fat lies about how we were injured, like telling new staff that I was caught in an elephant stampede. We just had to laugh at ourselves. Even a new quad learning to eat with his hand splint was funny to us.

Quads would team up with paras to get things done, passing on useful things we learned with an extraordinary sense of camaraderie. We were there for each other when our families just couldn't get this unique perspective we shared. When one of us said, "I understand," we could be sure he did. We gave each other some sense of normalcy in our lives, but sooner or later reality would rise to the top and all the anger, frustration, and uncertainty would erupt. One day I cried for hours under the weight of all the unknowns I was facing. The next day I was fine like nothing had happened. We were our own therapy group, keeping each other's spirits up, acting like the teens we were, but learning how to trust what we were feeling.

At last my name appeared on the blackboard in the nurse's station where they wrote the discharge dates — which we kept a close eye on. I was so happy to be through with therapy and felt that I had the knowledge and the skills I would need to move on. At the same time I was sad to be leaving my new friends.

In the ride home with Mom, my stepdad, and Julie in the VW van, I don't remember what we talked about — only that I was extremely happy to be going home. And then there we were in the driveway. My stepfather wheeled me in the house, and I was flooded with emotion, so happy to be back with my family, my room, and my things. I felt safe.

Since my injury, my friends were wishing me well, and being with them again was a big part of how I wanted to get back into my life. I went to a few parties, and the room would slowly empty when I came in. I didn't really notice it until it happened a few more times, and then I was shocked and very angry — in fact, devastated. I confronted a group at a party and said, "It's still me!" They could only stare down at the floor, saying nothing. Most of them I never saw again. I realize now that I reminded them of what could happen even to an invincible eighteen-year-old, and it was too uncomfortable for them.

I wanted to be part of a group again, so I spent my time with the only friends who stuck with me — Frank and his brother Bob. The local stoners. They and their friends welcomed me with open arms. They didn't care about the chair.

But I realized that if I wanted to get anywhere I had to go back to school. I had no real goals, but wanted to show my family I was going to keep moving forward. That helped keep me going through the tough times that were still ahead.

I eventually took or smoked every drug I could find and started doing dangerous things — taking chances that I knew were not smart. My attendant and I visited Mexico often, where we had a few close calls with the law but were never arrested.

One night my attendant and I were driving home after a heavy night of drugs and I said, "I want you to do exactly what I tell you, don't think, just do it." He was stoned enough to do it. I just wanted to see if my number would come up. I thought, "What could happen? I'm already a quad." So I told him how to drive, directing him to zip in and out of traffic on the freeway. We were passing a bus on the left shoulder when an overpass came up too fast as the shoulder narrowed. If the bus driver hadn't seen us, we would have become part of Interstate 5.

I decided to move out of the house with my attendant, one of the biggest reasons being that it was too hard on my parents to take care of me. Moms want to fix things when their kid is hurt, and this time she couldn't and it was overwhelming her. The best thing was to move out on my own.

My new place became party central with lots of girls, drugs, and more risk taking. Until the night when I was out with friends and got a call that my aide had overdosed on my Valium. He lived, but it was clear that it was time to get a grip on my life. One day I just said, "I can't do this anymore," and stopped taking drugs after almost eighteen years.

Amazingly, I stayed in school during all of this. I got my degree in psychology mainly because I wanted to get a grip on what I was going through. When the anniversary of my injury came around I would feel agitated and angry for days before and after. Over the years I often wondered why was I still alive and Del was dead. I wondered which of us was the lucky one. Years later I found out I was suffering from Post-Traumatic Stress Disorder. I was suffering from survivor guilt. Once I understood the problem, it was easier to deal with. I could recognize where my reactions and choices were coming from.

I also realized how my whole family and friends were affected by what had happened to me. I saw how I was so wrapped up in myself that I didn't see their pain, suffering, and frustration. I saw how my little sister Julie was neglected because of all the focus on me, yet Julie has stood by me the whole time. After all of this experience and time, my family has been able to talk about our feelings, and we have mended our relationships.

James — my best friend and one of my first aides — talked me into taking an "awareness training." Despite my resistance, I saw how it changed him, and it turned out to be just what I needed. It helped me focus even more on the issues I had been struggling with. I began volunteering at a skilled nursing facility, organized a few support groups, and visited the hard cases. In time a temporary position became a permanent job. I've worked now as a peer counselor for over twenty years. I've been able to use all of this life experience and the relationship and problem solving skills I've learned so I can help others.

Don Bondi lives in Aliso Viejo, California, where he works as a recreation director at a rehab and long term care facility. He's been an advocate for disability rights for thirty-four years, a peer counselor in independent living skills for twenty-five years, and is a member of the board of directors of the Dayle McIntosh Center for Transitional Living. Don reads science fiction, plays chess, builds models, and collects Egyptian artifacts.

My Body Is Only One Part of Me

Ginger Lane
C6-7
Age at SCI: 44
Date of SCI: February 23, 1984
Highland Park, Illinois

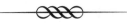

*I*never had the luxury of denial. The day after I hit a tree skiing, my father, a neurosurgeon, flew to Colorado. "How does it look? Is it permanent?" I asked. "Yes, it's permanent. You crushed your vertebrae at C6-7."

"But, how do you know it's permanent? My surgeon says I have a lot of swelling, and when it goes down, he'll be better able to tell," I wailed. My dad looked me in the eye and said kindly, "I've been practicing medicine for forty-seven years. I just saw your X-rays. I know."

I trusted my dad. After a long pause, I said, "But how will I live, what will I do, will I be in bed the rest of my life, what about my husband, my kids?" My fears, my confusion, and my anger came rushing out. Then, he answered, "After you get back home and are stable, you'll go to a rehabilitation hospital. You'll have to work hard to get stronger, to learn how to feed, bathe, and dress yourself, sit yourself up and use a wheelchair, and become productive again. Things will be different, but you'll live a life of dignity."

That talk was hard for me, even harder for him. No wishful thinking; no "I'll walk out of here." It's been eighteen years. Occasionally, I still wonder, "What would I be doing today if I hadn't hit that tree a million years ago?"

Did I have a choice in how to live my life? Yes, but it wasn't always apparent. I worried that my life would be determined by my quadriplegia, that I would have to define myself by my disability.

At first, it was hard — but made easier by a loving, supportive family, many friends, and good care. While lying completely immobilized on my rotating bed, I had a lot of time to think. Due to complications, I spent three months in acute care and four more in rehab. While it seemed like an eternity, it gave me the chance to work through some complex issues.

I had time to feel, to cry, and to examine a lot. From "How could I have missed that simple turn?" and "Did that tree have my name on it?" to "Will I ever sit up again or leave my bed?" and "Okay, stuff happens, but what do I do now?" In acute care, I was told that rehab would be like boot camp — if I didn't work hard enough, I'd get kicked out. And, if I didn't meet my insurance company's improvement rate, rehab couldn't justify my staying. I got scared, but motivated.

I stopped seeing my injury as the worst thing that could have happened; but, rather as an opportunity or challenge — to examine and re-focus my priorities and to grow. I remembered an article by psychologist Shere Hite examining why some people were able to come though difficult life changes successfully. She found that if they had negotiated a tough time early in life, they developed good coping skills that they could draw on as adults. The article resonated with me when I had first read it because of my background — living my early childhood in Berlin during World War II, losing my mother to Auschwitz, and being adopted by an American family, but having to give up my birth siblings. Since I'm pretty resilient, I decided that the best thing for me, as far as this awkward new body was concerned, was to learn about my body and work to regain and strengthen what physical function I could — not to wallow in self-pity.

I felt my world had drastically changed and shrunk, and I felt isolated, emotionally removed from my family and friends. Activities I loved —

dancing, skiing, playing tennis, bike riding, cooking — I could no longer do, at least not in the same way. When a recreation therapist wanted to talk, I refused. Then, angry and feeling sorry for myself, and hoping to get him to leave me alone, I told him, "I really want to ski down that mountain again" — thinking it would stump him. He pulled out a sports magazine. On the cover, a guy, sitting in what looked like a little covered sled, was skiing. He told me the skier had quadriplegia, like me. That motivated me to try skiing. I enjoyed it for about three years. But, it was always cold.

Dance became frustrating too. As a professional choreographer, I could no longer teach by demonstrating, and I didn't think I could perform in a wheelchair. I needed to shift into less physically demanding activities. This was very disappointing because dance was my first love. But, I kept reminding myself about that article and being resilient, and needing to move forward rather than longing for what used to be. It was time to start setting new goals.

One goal was to appreciate some of the little accomplishments I had made, like being able to raise my arm to scratch my nose or wipe away some tears, or actually get a forkful of chicken into my mouth by myself and not have someone else doing it. In the early stages, my focus was often on the big things, like walking. I needed to remember the important smaller things.

After seven months, I returned home. To solve the architectural issues, I moved into the first floor library, and we converted a "half bath" (sink and toilet) into a full bath by tiling the whole room and installing a hand-held shower. In my shower chair, I wheeled in backwards over the toilet, turned on the shower, and brushed my teeth at the tiny sink.

Harder to figure out was what to do with my increasing feelings of isolation. In rehab, I had felt "normal" — we were all disabled. It was our families who were different. With my new friends, I could cry, laugh, and complain — they understood. Psychotherapy then, and again later on, helped with my feelings of isolation, difference, and loss.

A friend connected me with a skier who'd become quadriplegic. Although I was apprehensive about calling her, when I did, I realized she was just like me. She knew how I felt because she had felt the same way. She validated my feelings and what I was going through and made me feel okay. She was my equal, a peer that I could trust and believe much more than my doctors or therapists because they hadn't experienced what I was going through. I felt understood and accepted. This was my first experience with peer counseling, and I valued it tremendously. She helped me because she had already gone through what I was experiencing, whereas my rehab friends were still in the same process I was in. She had perspective, we did not.

Not everyone has the chance to hook up with someone with whom they can identify so closely. I only talked to her twice. Then I found others who, although they hadn't had ski accidents, had gone through the same emotions of disbelief, shock, frustration, confusion, and then an eventual coming to terms, or accommodation, in order to integrate the changes into their lives. I also felt close to a rehab nurse who told me about her struggles going through a divorce and possibly moving and her child who was the same age as one of mine. Because we had so much in common, we commiserated together.

I didn't feel anger so much as sadness about the losses I needed to grieve: physical function, a sense of control over my life, independence, my established role in life, privacy, and my old sexual functioning. I also felt alienated from my own body. Once I identified my losses, I was able to grieve. I cried; but, at the beginning, I kept things to myself because I thought that expressing emotions was a sign of weakness. But, keeping everything inside wasn't working. As I started talking to others and expressing my emotions about feeling sad, lonely, and odd, I actually felt better. Now, I realize that sharing my thoughts and feelings was a sign of strength.

Going through the grieving process helped me grow, take a new direction, and realize that life does go on. I didn't need to feel so alone; support was available. With psychotherapy, I discovered I was really okay, could still like myself and my altered body and eventually reintegrate with my family, circle of friends, and community — and return to work.

Time was also important. I learned not to be in such a hurry trying to make things better — just to let them happen naturally. Things tend to take care of themselves and healing occurs. I began to appreciate that a body is just a body and not the totality of a person. I really began to like my body.

I have also become more introspective. I take more time to enjoy things and people — and to just be. I spend time examining my own life, and I enjoy helping others examine theirs.

Part of that process was dealing with my concerns around sex, desirability, body image, and self-identity. My husband and kids were really helpful by letting me know I was still a member of our family. Together, we learned that I was still who I was before the accident: a mom my kids could depend on for comfort and advice and still interested and involved in their school and social activities. And I was still a wife and partner to my husband. My identity was defined by who I was on the inside, not the condition or shape of my body or how well I could cook, garden, type, or dance.

While in rehab, on a field trip to an independent living center, I was surprised that most of the staff were disabled. Yet, I couldn't really identify with any of them or think that I might benefit from attending a support group there. I kept my distance, buying into the stereotypes about people with disabilities — unable to determine their own lives, helpless and dependent, not smart, unable to be productive — not realizing that I had some biases and prejudices, and was uncomfortable identifying myself as a disabled person.

Over the next few years, I started exploring some possibilities. First, I went on an overnight trip with two disabled friends. We helped each other, and it was fun discovering ways to make things easier for ourselves. Then, I started taking longer, more adventurous trips — an Alaskan cruise, a safari in Africa, and a month in Indonesia. Every challenge seemed to bring forth a creative solution. Asking for a second, but thin, mattress brought one bed in Africa up to a better height for transferring. Wheeling backwards got me out of a shower that dropped down from the rest of the floor. Discovering new tricks — using my arm rest as a reacher or my removable side guard as a sliding board — made me feel more confident and self-assured. When I got tired pushing up a hill, I turned around and started pulling backwards — working my biceps instead of my weaker triceps.

My inner journey of discovery had begun. I started to define myself not so much by what I did as by what I thought and felt. The more I felt comfortable in my own skin, the more I was able to say, "I am who I am — no matter what others think." The more I came to terms with my disability, the more I saw the possibilities available to me.

I went back to school and got a job providing psychosocial counseling to other disabled folks at the independent living center I had once thought had nothing to offer me. And, I became an activist. Some colleagues and I went to Washington and got arrested marching and demonstrating for passage of the ADA. Back home in Chicago, I became involved in starting a center focusing on the reproductive health and wellness needs of women with disabilities.

Becoming active in the disability rights movement and fighting for inclusion of people with disabilities into mainstream society has helped me with my self-identity as well as to recognize that I have strong convictions and a sense of purpose — with or without my disability. While my disability does not define the totality of who I am, it is an important part of me. To deny its presence is to deny an essential part of who I am — with all its attributes and limitations.

I no longer see the anniversary of my accident as a time to mourn. It's a time to acknowledge and celebrate the best in me and realize that it's always been there. I just had to find my own way to it. I like the course my life has taken, because it's really the course I chose. It's an ongoing process, a journey, and an opportunity to keep exploring and expanding my horizons.

Ginger Lane lives in Highland Park, Illinois. Six grandchildren keep her busy when she's not at work as peer counseling coordinator and disability rights advocate at Access Living, an Independent Living Center in Chicago. She is on the board of the Rehabilitation Institute of Chicago, chair of the Health Resource Center for Women with Disabilities, and a dancer with Dance>Detour, a company of dancers with and without disabilities.

Mourning and Healing

Daniel H. Gottlieb
C5-6
Age at SCI: 33
Date of SCI: December 20, 1979
Philadelphia, Pennsylvania

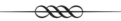

O n December 20, 1979, I kissed my wife and little girls goodbye, walked across my frozen lawn, and climbed into my brown 1976 Ford Mustang. While I was driving on the turnpike several hours later, a tractor-trailer going in the opposite direction lost its rear wheel. The wheel bounced across the turnpike, crushed my car, and severed my spinal cord. From that moment, I could neither move nor feel anything below my chest.

When I was taken to the hospital, I shouted, "Get me out of pain or kill me!" — referring to the emotional pain more than physical. I didn't really want to die; I wanted understanding and relief. I was in agony. People spoke to me differently and didn't make eye contact with me. My sense of alienation was terrifying.

Reassurances that I would "be okay" were no comfort. Relief came only when people had the courage to sit with me as I struggled to voice my confusion and figure out what of me had died and who I was now. I was fortunate enough to have family, friends, and a therapist who were courageous enough to listen to my painful story without giving me advice.

In those first several months, I wished only for death and relief from this terrible nightmare. My commitment to my young daughters was the only thing that kept me alive from day to day. My younger daughter had said, "Daddy, I'm glad you weren't hurt worse in the accident." I asked, "Why?" because I didn't particularly care whether or not I was hurt worse. She answered, "Because now I have my Daddy." I began to cry. I don't know why I cried. From that moment, I knew suicide was not an option.

But that's not the only reason why I didn't commit suicide. Weeks after the accident, I was morbidly depressed — even though I had an enormous support system of family and many friends. Having been readmitted to the Intensive Care Unit, I was in a halo vest with catheters and IVs connected to me. I was staring at the ceiling, contemplating what it would be like to be dead. I didn't know if I could go on. I didn't know if I wanted to.

A nurse came up to me and asked, "You're a psychologist, aren't you?" And I said, "Yeah." She asked, "At some point in their lives, do most people feel suicidal?" Since she didn't know that I was suicidal, I assumed she was talking about herself. I said, "It's not unusual. If you want to talk about it, after your shift, you can." Later, she came back and pulled a chair up next to my bed. With the halo vest, I couldn't see her face and didn't know who she was. After she told me about her life, I referred her to a psychotherapist I knew. That night, I knew I could live with my disability. She saved my life — by asking something of me.

In March 1980, I went to Magee Hospital for rehabilitation. At the end of each day, I remember how I would sit in my wheelchair looking out a picture window onto Race Street. I felt nothing but bitterness and envy toward everyone who walked or drove by. Even the homeless man sleeping on the vent on the corner didn't escape my bitterness. "At least he can get up and walk away if he wants to," I remember thinking. I believed that nothing could be worse than quadriplegia — nothing.

Today, I envy no one. My envy of others began to diminish as my "new" life developed. When people first started asking for advice and consultation, I began to realize that I had value.

I began to create a new life in rehab. At some level, I learned that I had the skills to do it. I also had good medical care, and that's terribly important. I especially valued the medical professionals who made eye contact with me, told me about their frustration with me, or shared a bit about their lives and their own sense of helplessness.

Late one night, a medical resident walked by my hospital room on his way home. He looked at me, stopped, and said, "You know, I have no idea what it is like to be you. But, my wife just had a miscarriage, a baby we very much wanted. If your pain is anything like mine, it must be awful." And he walked away. That was twenty-four years ago, and I still remember it. That was good medicine because in any trauma, people lose a sense of their own humanity and what it means to be human. I did, and I think everybody does. By looking me in the eye and saying, I don't know if your pain is like my pain but I got it, he affirmed that we were both people. I'm not a cripple and you're not a walker — we are people.

After I was in the hospital a few weeks, they were trying to strengthen my arms by putting me up on this piece of equipment where my arms were suspended with long springs — I looked almost like a marionette. With the springs, my arms were supported and I was turning pages in a book. Every day, the therapists reduced the support a little bit in order to build up my muscles. By the end of the week, I was able to turn the pages without any support at all. The occupational therapist said, "Dan, that's great. Aren't you proud of yourself?" I started to cry. I said, "You want me to be proud that I can turn a page. Two years ago, I wrote a three hundred and fifty page doctoral dissertation. How can I be proud of turning a page?" Then, in my mind, I was not yet a quad — I was an able-bodied man who couldn't turn a page.

When I first became quadriplegic, I would get very upset when I dropped something on the floor, needed help with my food, or was fatigued. I would feel angry, embarrassed, and sorry for myself. Yet, a few years later at a restaurant, I noticed that I was quite comfortable asking a friend to cut my food. Wondering what had created this change, I realized that for the first two years, my mind still believed I was an able-bodied man who was clumsy or lazy. But, at some point, the Dan Gottlieb I thought I was had died. Somehow, without noticing, I had become a quadriplegic.

My dreams reflected the process going on inside me. For the first two or three years after the accident, I dreamed of myself as able-bodied. When I woke up, I was either depressed or angry because of what I woke up to. Then, slowly but surely, I dreamed of myself as having minor infirmities, like I was able-bodied and strong but with no sensation in my hands. Or I was sitting in a wheelchair, but I didn't really need to because I was faking it. Gradually, the infirmities got more severe. But I never dreamt of myself as a quadriplegic. I believe that my mind was trying to figure out what was happening to me. At some point, there was a transition when my conscious mind said, "Now I get it, I'm a quadriplegic."

I lost Dan Gottlieb as I had known him for thirty-three years. I had to mourn the death of a future in which I would play golf and racquetball and be powerful and graceful. I also lost the trust that I would be safe in a benevolent world. I shed many tears over these losses. But, I gained the opportunity to be comfortable as a vulnerable man.

My values and my personality hadn't died — they were still here. But, in many respects, there had been a formidable death that needed to be grieved. To this day, I mourn for my losses. Not that I cry and feel sorry for myself everyday — just every now and then. This past spring, as I was driving to work by the river, I watched a couple jogging, and I just burst into tears — what I wouldn't give to be jogging with somebody I loved by the river on a spring day. I had to pull over, I was crying so hard. I cried for five minutes and then I went to work. All death must be mourned or it lays entombed inside of us forever.

I believe that my own mourning didn't set in for a year, at least. Initially, I was trying to recover from a trauma, physically and emotionally. My learning curve was pretty steep — I was busy learning how to be a quad.

I learned more about the healing process several years later when I was terribly depressed and despondent. I was dealing with a decubitis ulcer, my wife had left me, my children were at college, and my sister was diagnosed with a terminal illness. I was alone. I went to my doctor. He examined me and said, "It's broken," referring to my skin. I said, "I know," referring to my heart. Then he said, "Too much pressure." And I said, "I know." He continued,

"When a wound is moist, it is weeping (that's the jargon for a moist wound)."
I said, "I know."

After he cleaned my wound, he said, "You have to go to bed for about
thirty days." I asked, "How do you know?" He responded, "It's about three
centimeters, and wounds to the skin heal at a rate of about one millimeter a
day if the environment is clean." Then, when he said to cover it with this
brown substance, I said, "I thought it needed oxygen to heal. Why cover it?"
He said, "It does need oxygen to heal. But the oxygen it needs to heal comes
from your blood and not from the air. Everything your wound needs to heal
is already in your body. We just have to keep the environment clean and let
the body heal itself."

Wounds to the mind and the spirit are the same. My job as a psychotherapist is to keep the wound clean and get out of the way — knowing that
the wound is going to heal itself. My job is to have faith in the process — faith
in the life force, faith in the human psyche. That's my job — to keep it clean.
Things like judgment harm the wound. When we judge ourselves — I'm this
or I'm that — it does not keep the wound clean. Lots of things keep the wound
clean and help healing — being surrounded with love, not judging others, not
being with people who judge you, being in a context when you can help others. Given an environment of support, respect, and safety, more often than not,
the human spirit will heal itself.

During that same time of adversity and despair, I discovered a spiritual
dimension of my life that has also contributed to my healing. Because of the
ulcer, I was at home, in a bed, seeing patients. I was alone in the house other
than when people came to visit. After a while, I just stopped feeling alone. I felt
a kind of spiritual, divine companionship that I hadn't felt before. It is the kind
of companionship I have longed for all my life. It protects me from existential
loneliness. This divine companionship, this divine entity, only asks one thing
of me — faith. And, it only promises one thing — companionship. I don't feel
protected from any adversity. I don't feel protected from poor judgment. I don't
feel protected from anything. But when my heart is open and my faith is stable, I don't feel alone.

I am thankful that my doctors were honest enough to tell me that there was virtually no hope that I would ever walk again. When people tell me there is promising research in spinal cord injury, I smile and say, "Keep me posted," while I resist the seduction of hope. Hope can drain one's energy and interfere with the normal and healthy process of mourning losses.

I attribute part of the quality of my life to hopelessness! I was told there was no hope for a cure, and I believed it. After a period of severe depression, I began looking for a way to find happiness in a wheelchair. I never had hope that I could walk, but I always had hope that I would be happy.

Personally, hope scares me to death. I built my life, I like my life, and I see talk of a cure on the horizon as an expectation that my life could change radically again. I wouldn't say no, but I sure wouldn't be the first one in line. I'd get there when I got a break in my schedule.

Dan Gottlieb is a family therapist who lives and works outside of Philadelphia. In addition to his practice, he hosts a radio show on public radio, writes a column in the Philadelphia Inquirer, *speaks to a variety of audiences on healing, and relishes being a new grandparent.*

Transitions from the Abyss

Axel Doerwald
T11
Age at SCI: 37
Date of SCI: December 12, 1999
Mississauga, Ontario

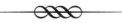

*H*as it really been three years already? Three years of toil to forge my new existence in this world as a disabled person. At times, it seems like only yesterday that I was walking down a stony path in the forest next to our new house, my children in tow, lock step behind me, moaning about sore legs and feet. Me, the drill sergeant, trying to muster up the troops for the long trek through the woods to the promised picnic site, "the troops" being two battle-weary girls under four years of age beseeching me for their lunch. These hikes were what I lived for and the reason we had decided to buy the house nestled gently in the midst of a forest with plenty of rugged trails on either side.

A few weeks later, after a nice dinner at home with friends, four of us decided to venture out on a night hike. Against our better judgment, we opted to trek towards the bluff in the opposite direction from where I had been with the kids. The icy December conditions, the darkness, and the presence of only a single flashlight portended disaster, yet we did not heed the warning signs.

A few days later, recuperating after seven hours of surgery, I was lying in the hospital bed, retracing a thousand times every one of what would turn out to be my final few steps in that darkness. I pondered incessantly and incredulously over the carelessness that led me to slip and fall off an eighty-foot cliff at night. I had hiked that trail more than a dozen times, both in the day and at night. Even with the morphine drip coursing through my veins, I was in bewilderment at my stupidity.

I remember the intern saying something about a fracture/dislocation at T11, spinal fusion, rods, squished spinal cord. Too much for me to absorb, so I thought of my wife and kids. They would be with me still. We could still live together, hug each other, laugh together, console one another. Couldn't we?

Where were they? I wanted them with me right in that moment. And then they were, running all over the room, asking a million questions, jumping on the bed, looking out the window, perusing my leftover hospital food with the anticipation of an unexpectedly found meal. I was in awe. To the kids, this was all a temporary respite from day-to-day life. Dad would be out in a matter of days, running with them, throwing them over his shoulder so they could ride high, wrestling with them. All would be back to normal.

Then a few days after — a sunny day in late December — I was alone, staring intermittently out the window, hearing children clambering all over the swings in the park below. I glanced back down at my legs as I had forty times in the last hour. They were still red and dormant, glistening a little. When I reached down to touch them, they seemed to belong to someone else. How strange. How will I ever get used to that?

Prior to my injury I lived anything but a sedentary lifestyle. I traveled often for business, exercised regularly, and loved hiking, camping, and the great outdoors. Immediately following my injury, my thoughts revolved around all the things that I could no longer do, the toys I could no longer use. Like my new mountain bike sitting silently in the garage, waiting to be ridden.

Looking back now, lying in that hospital bed after my operation with Christmas a mere week away was the hardest time of my life. While many tough roads lay ahead that I could not yet imagine, the first few weeks of realization were by far the hardest.

To cope, I thought constantly of my wife and kids. I tried to focus on the things we could still do together, the experiences we could still have. It was hard to envision, but I had to try and focus on the positives or I could feel myself sinking into depths of despair. I thought about the fact that I was alive. The miracle of it. Falling such a distance into a ravine of rocks and logs and surviving.

I went at my rehab with a vengeance, starting it just a few days after my surgery. I wanted to get out of the hospital and home to my wife and kids. Back to work running my business. In short, I wanted my old life back. I was home for a few days for a subdued Christmas season, everyone feigning gaiety around me. I remember having a hard time adjusting to my perceived inactivity. All around me, people were ambling about getting themselves drinks or food, cleaning up, preparing meals, etc. I just sat there and watched them all like a bump on a log. For someone used to hyperactivity as a normal course of affairs, this sedentary kind of lifestyle was hard to take.

I had been coming home every Friday starting a few weeks after the accident. On Sundays, my wife and kids would bring me back to the hospital. This was the worst time for me — to see them all walk out the door of my room, listening to the excited chatter of those two little girls as they shuffled down the hall. They were always sure to tuck Dad into bed for the night before they left. I lay there wanting to cry, prone again, listening to their voices recede into the distance, my mind paralyzed as much as my body was. At times like this, television offered a welcome escape from the unending turmoil that filled my thoughts.

About three months after my accident, I was discharged from rehab. In the first months, while I was busy researching new adaptive equipment, exercise and athletic options, running my business, and generally exploring my new world, it became increasingly apparent that my wife was having difficulties coping with the massive change that had been imposed upon us so suddenly. I sensed she was retreating further and further into a morass of despair.

Her escapist tendencies became more frequent and pronounced. I grew hostile and impatient with what felt to me like an ongoing rejection of what I had become. It slowly dawned on me that during rehab most of the focus was on me, my wife hearing repeatedly that she had to be strong for us both.

She had to "be there" for me like at no other time in our lives. While everyone who made those statements had the best intentions and were sincere in their advice, they missed the mark. No one was acknowledging her feelings and the demands of such profound changes in her life.

Now some two-and-a-half years later, the net effect is that our problems have spiraled massively out of control. It seems fairly evident to all concerned that the marriage cannot be salvaged. Why did this happen? Could it have been prevented? I ask myself these questions every day. What could I have done differently? I would alternate between consoling her for a few days, and when I saw nothing changing I would lash out and threaten divorce. She refused to consider counseling, so I felt she wasn't trying. For her though, counseling was for weak people who couldn't cope. We were strong individuals and had a strong relationship that had already survived numerous hardships. Or so we thought.

I felt I had moved on very quickly, re-establishing my life the best way I could. I was active in numerous physical activities, seeking to increase the number of things I could do. I bought a handcycle so we could all go riding together and an all-terrain chair so we could go in the forest or go camping together. Learning how to mono-ski was next on my list.

Everything I did was geared to getting back to my family and being able to participate with them in whatever we chose to do. I deeply resented that my wife was not joining me on this new journey, that I was going it alone without her support and reassurance. This caused me to falter. I started to experience feelings of futility. I started thinking to myself, "Well, if she doesn't want me, then no woman will. I am doomed to a life of celibacy, living alone in some squalid apartment, everything lost, waiting for my next disability payment."

I thought of Christopher and Dana Reeve and how they seemed to be coping so much better than we were and yet his functional loss was so much greater than mine. Why couldn't my wife be more like Dana? How was I failing to be supportive for her? Some of my actions were clearly not helpful. I felt alienated and relegated to the dust heap as a sexual being and lashed out at her as a result. A counselor once told me that when sex is present in a relationship it accounts for ten percent of the relationship in weighting of importance. When it is absent though, it counts for ninety percent. I felt that's what happened to us.

It became increasingly important for me to determine where I sat in terms of intimacy. It was like I had to prove to myself one way or another if women would still be interested in me. If it was really all over on that score, then I wanted to know right away. I started seeing other women that I met in bars or through the Internet. I told my wife that I was engaging in this, hoping she would come to her senses and take me back into her bed. She didn't. I found a number of other women that were very comfortable with me sexually and were keen to learn all my pleasure points and what activities I enjoyed. This was thrilling.

These women accepted me for who I was, dormant legs and all. They wanted to please me as much as I wanted to please them, they only needed me to show them how. I had learned something valuable from these experiences, having proved to myself that I was still capable of fulfilling a woman (and myself) in terms of intimacy. But what about my wife?

After two and a half years, we finally agreed to try counseling. But by this time, things had gone past the point of salvage. Both of us had been adulterous, and it seemed like nothing more could be done. Too much pain. Too much hurt inflicted by both parties. We had completely lost hope. The lesson learned was that early counseling was vital to our ability to weather the storm that disability brought to our relationship.

It is now three years later. I am starting a new chapter of my life as a single, disabled person and a divorced father of two beautiful little girls. Is it sad? You bet. I tell myself to hold out hope and eventually my life will get better. But why go there? Isn't the mere fact that I am alive to experience all the joys and sorrows and heartaches that life brings what matters? Isn't it as good now as it is ever going to get?

The unhappiest people I know are consumed by selfish desires. When I get depressed and try to analyze why I am feeling this way, the answer is very often that I relapsed into selfishness. The proverbial "Why me?" syndrome. Well, why not me? What makes me so special that I can escape the turmoil and struggle of daily life? The answer, of course, is nothing. When I consider things in these terms, I can better appreciate those aspects of life still available to me — even more than before my accident. The experiences I can still have hold greater weight and meaning than before, and I relish them all the more as a result.

Many people have talked to me about their feelings of futility and despair with their lot in life. So many tales of woe about money, jobs, spouses, and health issues. Then they turn to me and say, "Axel, you give me hope. If you can do it, so can I." How powerful is that? Here I am giving others hope and in so doing, giving myself hope as well.

The mind is the most notoriously difficult thing to control that I know of — with the notable exception of my bank account! How I perceive my life is really about what is going on in my mind. I do have the power to enforce positive change in my life. While I can't change all the circumstances around me, I can choose how I feel about them and how I react. And accept the transitions life brings.

Axel Doerwald lives in Toronto, Canada. He is recently separated and has two little girls named Kira (seven) and Reyna (six). He is the founder and president of Invatron Systems Corp., a successful software development house specializing in supermarket applications. He is an accomplished musician and spends his free time doing creative writing, skiing, and handcycling.

Teenager Interrupted

Erin Cornman
T11-12
Age at SCI: 13
Date of SCI: August 5, 2001
Carl Junction, Missouri

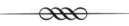

On the night of August 5, 2001, two days before my fourteenth birthday, I was in an automobile accident that broke my back, crushing my spinal cord at T11-12. I spent my birthday undergoing six hours of surgery to fuse my vertebrae together and stabilize my spine with titanium rods and pins. My injury was considered complete.

The following days in intensive care were a drug-induced blur until I was moved to a private room and had a constant stream of family and friends from school, church, and the community. Surrounded with cards, flowers, and gifts, my biggest concern at that point was being able to wash my hair! I still had no idea what had really happened and how my life would be changed. I believed I would soon be walking again, returning to life as usual.

There was no rehabilitation facility in our area with a pediatric doctor on staff, so we were forced to go somewhere far from home. My mom would be staying with me the whole time; my dad would have to commute, mostly on weekends. At this stage, I was in too much shock and didn't want to think about these details, so I left major decisions to them. Besides, I trusted them completely. So they chose Rusk Rehabilitation in Columbia, Missouri, five hours from home, which meant my dad could commute on weekends. Age has been both a blessing and a curse in my rehab. After reluctantly moving so far from home, my youth got me a big private room with a view. At Rusk, children and their families get top priority, enabling my mom and dad to sleep on a hospital mattress on the floor beside my bed.

We arrived with a mixture of high hopes and high anxiety, not really knowing what to expect. Within an hour of our arrival, a doctor crushed all hopes our family had for my recovery. He told us bluntly there was less than a five-percent chance I would ever walk again and that I probably would not live much past 60! I'm sure he believed that blunt honesty was the best thing for us, but we experienced him as cruel and without compassion.

And we knew better. My mother had already spent a lot of time on the Internet, thanks to a social worker in the hospital who found her a room where she could surf while I had visitors. She found research showing that people with spinal cord injury live longer, healthier lives than ever before. We'd also visited personally with two people who were injured in their twenties and were now in their late sixties and healthy.

So my mother confronted him and demanded he apologize. At first, he was shocked by the challenge to his authority, but then seemed genuinely sorry. Still, we requested a different doctor with whom we had a much better rapport. He was a young, pediatric specialist who had a son my age and a sense of humor, too!

The impact of what had really happened hit me hard in my first week at rehab while my mom was helping me into the shower. I wasn't able to transfer myself yet and didn't know that I'd be independent someday. As a teenager, I was already trying to break away from my mom, and now it felt like I was going to have to be treated like a baby for the rest of my life. I broke down crying saying, "I don't want to be paralyzed!" My mom broke down too, unable to stop my pain while she tried to reassure me that everything would be alright. I was mature for my age, both mentally and physically, and have always been a very independent, strong-willed person. Relying on someone else for my needs or having to do things I didn't want to do was unacceptable to me. Like a lot of teens, I thought I knew everything. Being forced back into dependence on my parents felt like a giant step backwards. I argued constantly, not wanting to be controlled by other people's rules. I couldn't see that the things they were asking me to do were for my own health. I felt like I was being deprived of my youth.

Now I realize I was just afraid of the unknown. Eventually, it became clear that staying healthy would require me to adopt some new daily routines, like morning stretches and taking medications. I realized that my injury didn't affect the most important part of who I am. The adults were not trying to dominate my life. By teaching me these techniques, they were helping me learn to be independent again. They wanted that for me as much as I did. I began intensive physical, occupational, and recreational therapy. My family and I were bombarded with information about spinal cord injury in daily classes. Being just a few weeks into my injury experience, it was still hard for me to care much about any of it. I was in a lot of pain and was trying hard to adjust, so it was difficult to participate in areas of therapy that didn't seem to pertain to me. Eventually I realized that my time in rehab was short, and I couldn't wait until I felt better to learn the things that were vital to my rehabilitation.

I knew I would not be allowed to go home until I reached a certain level of independence. And even though several friends made the five-hour trip to Columbia to visit me, I really missed them, and this added to my desire to work hard — along with the encouragement and persistence of my doctor, therapists and parents. This gave me the incentive I needed. Now I'm grateful for everything I learned in rehab. It has had a positive effect on my life. I'm putting that knowledge to practical use every day, customizing what I learned during rehab according to my needs.

The true test was going home, leaving the controlled environment of rehab, where everything was accessible and everyone had the same issues. We weren't sure what to expect, but imagined it would be difficult at first. I had to move out of my upstairs bedroom and into my parents' room. We soon learned we had to plan most of our outings around stairs, doorways, and bathrooms. But things started to improve gradually. Eventually, we purchased an accessible van and by trial and error we learned where I could and couldn't go. Fortunately, we discovered that the places I could go far outnumbered the places I could not.

Before the accident, I was a freshman starting high school, excited about all the new social opportunities and freedom I would gain. However, going in a wheelchair was not quite what I had envisioned. I was really worried that people my age might think I wasn't capable of doing things with them anymore. I was afraid they would stop including me socially.

Instead of having more freedom, I was spending nearly all of my time with my mom, who was my primary caregiver. Instead of my days being filled with teenage girl things, they were filled with therapy, doctor's appointments, tutoring, sickness, and fatigue. But most of the kids at school were supportive, and the teachers and faculty went out of their way to be helpful — much to my relief.

My overall health improved and my strength and stamina began to return. This meant less time at the doctor and more freedom from my mom! Finally, I no longer required a tutor and was able to go to school full time. I was back in the same routine as everyone else, much more accepting of my situation. Even though the accident didn't happen to my friends and family, it affected their lives too. At first, they didn't always know what to do or how to act. Some of my "friends" couldn't handle my injury and it didn't take long to figure out who they were. It hurt me, but you can't force someone to be your friend. To me, it separated the shallow people from the more mature, compassionate ones. I've learned what the important qualities are in people, besides how they look or how cool they are.

I've made new friends who love me for who I am now, not who I was before. I found that talking about my injury and answering all their questions puts them at ease. People are generally very curious. Knowing the facts instead of being left wondering makes all the difference. They want to know things like how I get dressed, take a shower, or get in and out of the car. It's always funny when people say, "Oh, okay ... well, that makes sense." It makes me wonder how they thought I did it! My school principal confided to my mom that in the first months after I was back, the teachers and staff were scared to death of doing something that might hurt me. Now they've asked their questions, have learned about SCI, and treat me like any other student — instead of a china doll.

It didn't take long to realize that I had two choices for my life. One was to feel sorry for myself and give up, or I could get on with it and make the most of what I had. Actually, I don't think I ever really considered the first option. Once the initial shock wore off and the reality became clear, I made up my mind. I was fourteen years old then with too much life ahead of me to be miserable by choosing option one. I knew what I wanted to do, but the problem was figuring out how to go about it.

So I started at the only place I could — the beginning — and took it one day at a time, driven by my determination and my parents' support. My mom is as strong-willed as I am, and there have been many days when we wanted to kill each other! But she never lets up, and I refuse to give up. People comment on my positive attitude and how happy I seem to be. We always wonder why they are so amazed about it. I just made a choice and never looked back.

Is life different now? Yes, but it's meaningful and I'm having a lot of fun. Would I be on this road if I'd had the choice? No, but this is my life, and I intend to make something of it. I don't dwell on things I can't do any-more. I focus on the things I can. I participate in concert choir, journalism, debate, voice lessons, tutoring elementary school children, church youth group, riding horses, swimming, babysitting, shopping, eating out, and going to the movies. At first, many of these activities seemed intimidating, either because I wasn't sure how I would do them or because it meant being around new people. But the first time is always the hardest. I do my best to plan well, but surprises still happen. It can be aggravating to have to take all the extra time and then have something still not work out. Adjusting to life with a spinal cord injury doesn't happen overnight. It requires patience, but it does happen.

My life will always be an ongoing process. Having a disability doesn't mean that I can't change things for the better. Finding acceptance doesn't mean giving up hope that they will continue to make progress with research. I plan to attend medical school when I graduate and who knows what I might be able to contribute someday? I have a great life now and a great plan for the future. I might have to take the longer road there, but I could have missed a lot along the way otherwise. Wish me luck on my journey!

Erin Cornman lives with her parents, Keith and Suzanne Cornman, and her dachshund, Sophie, in Carl Junction, Missouri, where she is a Junior at Carl Junction High School. She is active in concert choir, voice training, horseback riding, A+ tutoring, church youth group, and community volunteer work. She recently obtained her driver's license and works part-time at J.C. Penney. Erin's goal is to attend medical school and become a psychiatrist.

About the Editors

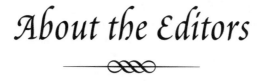

Gary Karp is the author of *Life On Wheels: For the Active Wheelchair User* (O'Reilly & Associates, 1999), and *Choosing A Wheelchair: A Guide For Optimal Independence* (O'Reilly & Associates, 1998), widely considered definitive guides for people with disabilities. He draws from his personal experience with spinal cord injury since 1973, when he was injured in a fall from a tree at the age of eighteen. His feature articles appear regularly in *New Mobility* magazine, he has written for a variety of disability-related Web sites, and he is a board member of the National Spinal Cord Injury Association, for whom he also writes a monthly column. He is also a guest commentator for "Perspectives" on KQED-FM, San Francisco's public radio affiliate. A popular international speaker, Gary is sponsored in part by the Christopher and Dana Reeve Paralysis Resource Center. He is also a consultant in computer ergonomics, a musician and a juggler, and lives in San Rafael, California, with his wife, Paula.

Stanley D. Klein, Ph.D., a clinical psychologist and frequent speaker to parents and health care and education professionals, has worked with children with disabilities and their parents for fifty years. In recent years, he worked with adults with disabilities as Education Director for Abilities Expo. A recipient of numerous national awards for his work, he was co-founder and former editor-in-chief of *Exceptional Parent* magazine. He has co-edited *The Disabled Child and the Family* (Exceptional Parent Press, 1985), *It Isn't Fair: Siblings of Children with Disabilities* (Greenwood Publishing Group, 1993), *You Will Dream New Dreams: Inspiring Personal Stories by Parents of Children with Disabilities* (Kensington Books, 2001) and *Reflections on a Different Journey: What Adults with Disabilities Want All Parents to Know* (McGraw-Hill, 2004). The father of two adult children, Stan lives in Gloucester, Massachusetts, is active in politics, and enjoys trying to play tennis.

Resources

National Organizations

National Spinal Cord
Injury Association
800-962-9629
www.spinalcord.org

American Association of
People with Disabilities
866-241-3200, www.aapd.com

National Council on
Independent Living
703-525-3406, www.ncil.org

National Organization on
Disability, 202-293-5960,
www.nod.org

Paralyzed Veterans of America
800-424-8200, www.pva.org

World Institute on Disability
510-763-4100, www.wid.org

Publications

Disability Studies Quarterly
www.afb.org/dsq/index.html

New Mobility
www.newmobility.com

Paraplegia News
www.pvamagazines.com/pnnews/

Ragged Edge Magazine
www.raggededgemagazine.com

SCI Life
www.spinalcord.org

Spinal Network: The Total
Wheelchair Resource Book
www.spinalnetwork.net

Sports N' Spokes
www.sportsnspokes.com

Information Resources

The Center for Research on
Women with Disabilities
800-44-CROWD
www.bcm.tmc.edu/crowd

Christopher and Dana Reeve
Paralysis Resource Center
800-593-7309, www.paralysis.org

The Christopher Reeve
Paralysis Foundation
800-225-0292, www.crpf.org

Disability Resources
www.disabilityresources.org

International Ventilator
Users Network
314-534-0475
www.post-polio.org/ivun/ivun

Miami Project to Cure Paralysis
305-243-6001
www.miamiproject.miami.edu

National Foundation for
the Treatment of Pain
831-655-8812, www.paincare.org

National Rehabilitation
Information Center
www.naric.com

The National Strategy
for Suicide Prevention
800-SUICIDE, www.mental
health.org/suicideprevention

North Carolina State
Center for Universal Design
800-647-6777
www.design.ncsu.edu/cud

Resources

The Spinal Cord Injury
Information Network
www.spinalcord.uab.edu

Assistive Technology

Abilities Expo
www.abilitiesexpo.com

Center for Assistive Technology &
Environmental Access (CATEA)
www.assistivetech.net

Employment

The Job Accommodation Network
800-526-7234, janweb.icdi.wvu.edu

Legal Rights

The Disability Rights Education
and Defense Fund
510-644-2555, www.dredf.org

Sexuality

www.Sexualhealth.com

Sports and Recreation

Disabled Sports USA
301-217-0960, www.dsusa.org

National Center on
Physical Activity and Disability
800-900-8086, www.ncpad.org

The Arts

The National Arts
and Disability Center
310-794-1141, nadc.ucal.edu

For Families

The National Family
Caregivers Association
800-896-3650, www.nfcacares.org

Religion

Religion and Disability Program
202-293-5960, www.nod.org/
religion

Travel

The Society for Accessible
Travel & Hospitality
212-447-7284, www.sath.org

Access-Able Travel Source
www.access-able.com

And ... do some surfin'.

www.adawatch.com
www.bentvoices.org
carecure.rutgers.edu/spinewire
www.concretechange.org
www.survivingparalysis.com
www.DisABILITIESBOOKS.com
www.halftheplanet.com
www.healingtherapies.info
www.ican.com
www.lifeonwheels.org
www.notdeadyet.org
www.sci-info-pages.com
www.makoa.org/sci.htm
www.sciwire.com
www.spinlife.com
www.wheelchairjunkie.com

OTHER TITLES AVAILABLE FROM THE PUBLISHER OF FROM THERE TO HERE

NEW MOBILITY
A hip monthly lifestyle magazine for wheelchair users, *NM* covers health, people, relationships, sex, parenting, work, art, recreation, travel, products, cure research and the all the tools you need to live life to the fullest.

SPINAL NETWORK: THE TOTAL WHEELCHAIR RESOURCE BOOK
Spinal Network is a 586-page resource book for wheelchair users that the *Los Angeles Times* calls "awesomely complete." It includes inspiring profiles of survivors; insider knowledge on functional return and cure research; opportunities for sports, recreation, travel and the arts; details on sex, fertility, pregnancy and parenthood; strategies for hiring, firing and managing personal attendants; features on finding the right wheelchair and other equipment; plain talk on complicated government benefits programs; resources for hundreds of organizations, and much more.

ENABLING ROMANCE
Enabling Romance is a guide to love and relationships for people with disabilities and the people who care about them. Packed with stories and practical information, this book reveals successful approaches for finding and maintaining love on wheels.

COMPLETE PRODUCT GUIDE FOR PEOPLE WITH DISABILITIES
The Complete Product Guide is a comprehensive reference book that describes more than 1100 disability products, and includes photos and full contact information. Essential for making informed buying decisions.

KIDS ON WHEELS
Kids on Wheels is a unique two-volume resource book. Vol. 1 is written for grade-school kids with disabilities and includes profiles of other kids, recreation opportunities and more. Vol. 2 is for parents and professionals, and covers everything you need to know to empower a child with a disability.